CRACKING

THE

CODE

OF THE

DIET

AND

FOOD

INDUSTRIES

SARENA S. JOHNSON

Order this book online at www.trafford.com
or email orders@trafford.com

Most Trafford titles are also available at major online book retailers.

Print information available on the last page.

ISBN: 978-1-4120-5054-8 (sc)

Trafford rev. 02/13/2020

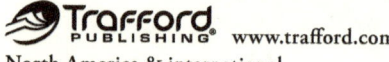 www.trafford.com

North America & international
toll-free: 1 888 232 4444 (USA & Canada)
fax: 812 355 4082

Acknowledgments

To God—the "Creator" of everything—including the healthiest foods available.

Then God said, "I give you every seed-bearing plant on the face of the whole earth and every tree that has fruit with seed in it. They will be yours for food" (Gen. 1:29, NIV).

To my husband and children, for all the hours of family time you gave up so Mommy could work on the "pewter."

To my friends and sisters for their input, inspiration, and friendship.

To you, for buying this book. I pray you will be motivated to change the actions that keep you in bondage so you may live the extraordinary life God planned for you and the ones you love.

Contents

APPENDICES

INTRODUCTION

T HIS BOOK IS about getting you the information you need to change your life. Knowledge is not power. Getting the correct information, learning how to apply that information, and taking action—that's power! Power is knowing that every action you make today will cause a reaction. You can decide to make positive healthy choices that make a difference. That is what this book is about. Empowering you, through education, motivation, and support to change your actions. This book is a first step in educating you with correct information.

Take note! Being healthy is not about living a perfect health-and-fitness lifestyle; it's about changing everyday actions, actions that will make an enormous difference in your life.

Your lifestyle is largely determined by what you are eating, if you are exercising, and other actions you choose throughout your day. We have a lot of choices every day. You may not understand all of them. That is why I am writing this book—to show you how to take control, change the way you look and feel, and dramatically improve the quality of your life.

Americans are not well. We are a very sick society. Most of us are walking "dead." We are dying from lack of motivation, oxygen, and energy; we are also experiencing an increase in physical illnesses and mental disorders. Here are some overwhelming facts. According to the Centers for Disease Control (CDC):

- More than 44 million Americans are considered obese. This reflects an increase of 74 percent since 1991.[1]

- Over 60 million people (a third of the population) are overweight.[2]

- The percentage of young people who are overweight has more than doubled in the last twenty years. Of children and adolescents aged 6–19, 15 percent—about nine million young people—are considered overweight.[1]

- Chronic diseases account for seven of every ten U.S. deaths and more than 60 percent of medical care expenditures. In addition, the prolonged illness and disability associated with many chronic diseases decrease the quality of life for millions of Americans.[3]

- More than 90 million Americans live with chronic illnesses.[3]

- Chronic diseases account for 70 percent of all deaths in the United States.[3]

- Cardiovascular disease (primarily heart disease and stroke), cancer, and diabetes are among the most prevalent, costly, and preventable of all health problems.[3]

Many of these chronic diseases are preventable. Physical inactivity and unhealthy eating contribute to obesity, cancer, cardiovascular disease, and diabetes. These two behaviors are responsible for at least 300,000 deaths each year. This can all be slowed down, prevented, or stopped by changing our unhealthy behaviors that increase our risk for chronic diseases.

It seems that every day we get hit with new information from the diet and food industries. More food choices, confusing "lingo," new diets—help! Help is here. You have a choice right now. You can continue on the same path— making the same choices, looking and feeling the same way, and living with the pain, hurt, and agony of your unhealthy actions—or you can decide to change, to take control of your life. You can make a difference in your life and the lives of those around you.

PART ONE:
CRACKING THE CODE OF THE DIET INDUSTRY

AMERICANS ARE SEEKING an easy solution to their weight problems. Of the 55 million Americans who go on a diet program only 5 to 10 percent succeed. Sad news for Americans, great news for the "diet industry". This "weight-loss" industry amasses an estimated 40 billion in revenue annually. By the year 2006, revenue is estimated to top 48 billion.[1]

In this section, learn how you can STOP becoming a "slave to the cycle" of dieting, depression, energy depletion, and sickness—and start living a life filled with energy and healthful abundance.

Potions, pills, diet food, and drinks—oh my! Don't be a statistic any longer. Get ready to "crack the code."

NOTES

"THE GREATEST TRAGEDY IS NOT DEATH, BUT LIFE WITHOUT PURPOSE."
—RICK WARREN, *THE PURPOSE DRIVEN LIFE*

1

What "They" Won't Tell You

WHAT YOU DO each day matters. Before you begin, you need to know that every action you take today has a consequence. It can either be positive or negative. Here are a few steps to make your actions work for you.

Decide to change. Questions to think about...

What actions control your life? (What do you spend most of your day doing?)

What are your priorities in life? (God, family, health, food, work, shopping)

What are your goals? (Determine your goals and spend each day contributing to them. See Appendix 2 "Actions Diary" for more.)

The fact is, we spend most of our day performing actions that have no purpose in our life. We watch hours of television, go shopping, and worry about everything we have to do. We spend our days being "active" but not "proactive." If you know what your purpose is, and what your goals are, you can spend the day being proactive and contributing to your purpose and goals. Below are tips to help you stay focused on your healthy lifestyle.

KEEP IT SIMPLE

It can be overwhelming to try improving your health all at once. Instead, focus on a few healthy actions you can add to your daily routine, such as eating more fruits and vegetables or walking. After a while, these new healthy actions will be routine and you can then concentrate on adding a new healthy action.

BELIEVE IT

There will always be reasons you can't do something if you don't believe you can. Don't focus on why you're not achieving your goal(s). (I can't find a sitter, there is no time, and I have a meeting.) Instead, make a list of actions (barriers) that are preventing you from living a healthy lifestyle; next to it, list an action (strategy) that will contribute to your healthy lifestyle (see Appendix 2 "Goal Form"). For example, if you eat "junk food" when you are stressed or bored, don't buy the junk (or throw it out—it's junk!). Replace those foods with fruits and vegetables. If it's not there it can't be eaten.

PRIORITIZE YOUR HEALTH

We all have the same number of hours in the day. We all have busy lives. There will probably never be a perfect time in your life to exercise and eat right because you don't have anything else to do. The truth is, taking care of yourself is a responsibility. When you put your health last, everything else suffers. It isn't doing you, your family, or your friends any favors if you are overweight, have high-blood pressure, are stressed out, and tired all the time. Schedule nutritious meals and exercise into your day.

CONCENTRATE ON THE POSITIVES

Instead of looking at exercising as one more thing you have to do, think about exercise as an hour of "me time." Instead of thinking about unhealthy food as "comfort food," try to associate healthy food with happy times. For example, think about how your body responded, both physically and mentally, when you ate a diet with plenty of fruits and vegetables (instead of high-sugar, high-processed foods). How did your body's positive response affect your attitude? How did this affect your day and the people around you?

Now that you are ready to change, turn to Appendix 2 "Logs & Forms" and fill out your Action Diary, Goal-Setting Form, Contract to Change, and Food Log. These forms will help you concentrate, visualize, and motivate you to your new healthy lifestyle.

NOTES

2

THE "IT" PRINCIPLE FOR SUCCESS:
WANT IT! THINK IT! BELIEVE IT! SEE IT! WRITE IT! PLAN IT! DO IT!

YOU HAVE TO want to change. Take action! Think about your goals (what you want to accomplish)— every day. Get visual aids or pictures of what your goals are. Write your goals down. Plan out what actions you will do each day to reach your goals. Play out those actions every day. Focus on the actions you need to take, not what you shouldn't do. For example, I am eating more fruits today in place of soda pop.

CHANGE YOUR FOCUS

One reason diets and goals fail is that individuals concentrate on what they shouldn't eat and what they shouldn't do. (If you can't have it, that is when you want it!) In addition, their mental focus is "I can't eat that." Change your focus. Focus on what you should do every day. Don't let the focus be food. Enjoy your food. Let it be God, family, exercise, and fun. Keep your goals in mind!

CLEAN YOUR HOUSE

After you have committed to take action start by throwing away all the "junk" food. Stock your house with fruits, vegetables, and whole grain products such as oatmeal, brown rice, and whole wheat pasta. Read ingredients and make sure products are 100 percent whole wheat or whole grain not just unbleached wheat.

GET SUPPORT

Accountability plays a large part in success. If you are feeling down or distracted a supporter can lift you up and motivate you to keep going. A supporter is also great to help you keep your exercise appointments!

SHRINK IT!

Studies have shown that when a person has a larger serving she will eat more. Instead of filling up all at once, use a small bowl or plate and go back for more. (You'll get more exercise too!)

GET SLEEP

Research has revealed that a good night of sleep is one of the most important elements in good health.

If we are tired it affects our exercise (we move less), our attitude (we're cranky), and our eating habits (we eat more).

DENSITY COUNTS

Emphasize foods with a low-caloric density (fruits, vegetables, and soups, which have lots of water), instead of high-calorie dense foods (chips, meats, cakes, doughnuts), which contain a high caloric value compared to their weight.

LIMIT CHOICES

This is the same concept as above. The more food choices you have the more you will eat. Cut out high-fat, highly-processed foods ("white" foods). Keep it simple with whole (minimally processed) foods such as grains, fruits, and vegetables.

KEEP MOVING

What you do matters. Just as those little calories in candy and condiments add up so do all the little activities you do. Walk, jiggle, and move when you can. Make sure you add cardiovascular (aerobic) activities and strength training too!

QUICK TIP

It takes about 3500 calories to lose or gain a pound. If you drink an "extra" beverage containing 140 calories and don't change your activity, you will gain 1 pound about every 23 days. That's almost 16 pounds a year!

If you exercise and burn an extra 140 calories a day—and your eating habits remain the same—you could lose those 16 pounds in one year!

NOTES

WHAT IS YOUR "WHY" FOR CHANGE? WHEN YOUR "WHY" IS STRONGER
THAN YOUR CURRENT SITUATION, THAT'S WHEN YOU CHANGE.

3

SLAVE TO THE CYCLE?

IF YOU HAD the choice to buy one of the following cars, which would you choose?

1. A car with all the bells and whistles, exhilarating to drive, looks better than your bed after a long work day, but has a lot of problems: a "poor" repair history, the air bag is known to explode at random, the steering wheel has a mind of its own, and it guzzles gas like drinking water.

or

2. A car that looks, "OK," has minimal "bells and whistles," and never gives you that "excitement" or "emotional high" from touching, seeing, and driving it. However, it's the best consumer rated car for repair

history and crash tests, lasts longer than the energizer bunny, and gives an astounding 40 mpg.

Most would choose car #2. Consumers like to get the most for their money. Why not get the most from your food?

If you had to choose from the following foods, what would you choose?

1. A food that looks better than water in the desert, tastes better than anything you've ever tasted, the smell causes you to drool, and the price is the greatest deal of the century. But if you ate this food, it would end up costing you more, make you sick, rob you of energy, starve your body, and make you fat at the same time. Would it be as appealing?

or

2. A simple food that looks "OK," tastes "OK," and has a neutral smell. When you eat it you have more energy, feel better than ever, lose weight, and your health improves.

The above scenarios correlate to a nutrient-deficient, high-fat, highly-processed American diet, and a nutrient-dense, whole foods diet. Most think they are getting a value when they buy a large quantity for a low price. Frequently, that turns out to be car #2 or food #1. It looks good, smells good, tastes good, but has numerous problems. It starves the body of nutrients, depletes our energy, and causes sickness and weight gain. You are really not getting a value at all!

One of the biggest problems I hear as a professional, and have faced myself, is what happens when the body always wants to eat because it is continuously given nutrient-deficient food. What happens? A host of problems. Nutrients are never acquired. Energy is lost. Sickness is frequent. Weight gain occurs and/or is kept. It's a nutrient-deficient roller coaster. You become a slave to the cycle.

You don't have to be a slave any longer! You have a choice to change today. Below are steps you can take to stop the cycle.

1. Eat whole foods all or most of the time. (Foods in their natural state which don't have a label or don't need one.)

2. Eat whole foods in their "raw" (uncooked) state, when possible (vegetables, fruits, seeds, and nuts).

3. Eat organic foods as often as possible.

4. Find out what your body likes and dislikes. Most importantly, notice how your body reacts (both mentally and physically) after you have eaten.

5. Consider the cost of the food you are about to eat. What is the cost in energy, mood, weight, and overall health? What will eating it now cost you later?

I have included a food log in Appendix 2 for you to write down the foods you eat and what they cost you in feelings and physical reactions. This is a useful tool in getting to know your body.

Don't drive yourself crazy trying to eat perfect. Try focusing on including foods in their natural state all or most of the time. In addition, remember, every body is different.

QUICK TIP

Stress such as that from sleep deprivation, work, and everyday family life takes a toll on our body systems, causing a weakened immune system. Our immune system is further damaged by poor eating habits, which leads us to more health problems. Stress often causes us to eat more carbohydrates for energy and the tranquility effect we get from tryptophan (which the body converts into serotonin.)

Combat stress with a good night's rest, supplements, and eating healthy tryptophan foods such as bananas, pineapples, avocados, tomatoes, eggplant, and walnuts.

NOTES

WHEN DIET IS WRONG MEDICINE IS OF NO USE.
WHEN DIET IS CORRECT MEDICINE IS OF NO NEED.
—ANCIENT AYURVEDIC PROVERB

4

FOOD LOVER,
CALORIE CUTTER

DO YOU LOVE to eat? I do! This is another benefit of whole foods.

You see, foods are not created equal. Nutrient-packed whole foods such as fruits and vegetables have fewer calories but fill you up! This is called calorie density. If you eat foods with low calorie density (which have lots of water) instead of high-calorie dense foods such as chips, meats, cakes, doughnuts, you can eat more—with added benefits!

Did you know that the fat content in one cup of whole milk equals twenty cups of green peas or eight cups of brown rice?

Now, I am not saying "eat no fat." The information above

is shown to give you a mental picture of differences in food. As stated in Chapter 2, these differences are not only in fat, but in the energy and quality of health they provide.

According to a report by the Center for Science in the Public Interest soft drinks are the fifth largest source of calories for adults, providing 5.6 percent of all the calories that Americans consume.[1] This does not stop at adults!

Boys age twelve to nineteen who consume soda pop drink an average of two 12-ounce sodas per day (868 cans per year). Girls drink about one-fourth less. Soft drinks provide the average 12- to 19-year-old male with about fifteen teaspoons of sugar a day and the average female with about ten teaspoons a day.

It's not just sugar in soda that has obesity on the rise. It can be the calories in juice or other beverages, the butter on the bread, the cream in the coffee, and candy that's eaten. Americans eat all the time! We eat to celebrate. We eat when we're sad, tired, or bored. We eat after church, we eat before church, we eat when we get up, we eat when we go to bed.

If you want to change your health, you need to change your food choices. Take notice of all the little "extras" you are putting in your mouth each day. Extras while you drive, while you eat, while you talk, while you cook, while you clean the plates off the table, while you set the plates on the table, and so on.

Again, benefits of whole foods are they fill you up, have fewer calories, and are packed with nutrients.

It is important to understand that individuals need different amounts of fat and calories depending on their activity level, body fat, muscle mass, etc. Calorie needs change from day to day. Don't expect to eat the same amount of calories every day. Some days you will exercise, work all day, cook, clean, dress your children, and run errands—and that's just the beginning. Other days may be less active. Like a child, listen to your hunger—listen to your body.

Finally, if you are trying to lower your body fat, you will need to concentrate on eating more of the low-calorie dense foods such as fruits and vegetables. In this case, I recommend that the majority of your daily food intake be fruits and vegetables, followed by whole grains (whole-grain brown rice, beans, and legumes), and seeds and nuts (in limited quantities).

You have a choice. What will you choose to do today?

QUICK TIP

In America, we tend to eat our biggest meal of the day at dinner—right before bed. This is not the case in other countries. Give your metabolism and body an energy boost throughout the day—and a rest at night (don't eat three hours before bed)—by eating your biggest meal of the day at lunch (or the first half of your day). This is the one of the greatest weight loss/maintenance "secrets."

NOTES

"IF CONFUSION IS THE FIRST STEP TO KNOWLEDGE, I MUST BE A GENIUS."
—LARRY LEISSNER

PART TWO:
CRACKING THE CODE OF THE FOOD INDUSTRY: BECOMING SUPERMARKET SAVVY

T HIS SECTION WILL help you navigate your way through the confusing labels, lists of ingredients, and nutrition information. Because ingredients and labeling are comprehensive, I have included many, but not all, terms associated with labeling and ingredients. Furthermore, because there are so many "codes" this is a great tool as a reference.

When shopping, remember, all foods in a "health food" store are not necessarily "healthy." This applies to foods made by the same manufacturer too. In addition, not all foods that are "natural" are good for you. Tobacco is natural and it has killed many people. Your best weapon is to read and understand food labels and ingredients.

5

CRACKING THE CODE OF LABELS

DO YOU FEEL like you're reading a secret code when reading a food label? Terms such as "Organic," "Lite," "Kosher," "Vegan," "Lactose Free," "Pareve," (or "Parve"). In addition, labels also contain symbols and letters! What do they mean?

To help you "crack the code" this chapter includes information on how to read food labels, what those label terms mean, and how they apply to you!

If your diet consists of a variety of good quality whole foods eaten when you are hungry, there is no need to frustrate yourself with figuring calorie intake, percentages, etc.—though it may be a good guide to estimate your nutrient intake.

Grab your grocery labels and read on!!

VEGETARIAN TERMS

Kosher is anything marked with the kosher symbol. There are about three-hundred kosher certified agencies in the U.S., and several different symbols. The most common symbols contain the letter "K," and the letter "U" with a circle. Kosher food is manufactured in accordance with Hebrew dietary laws, which state that dairy products cannot be combined with meat products. Therefore, the kosher symbol indicates that the product contains dairy or meat but not both.

Kosher Dairy is symbolized by the letter "D" alongside the "K" symbol. It indicates a product that contains dairy. The letters "DE" indicate it was produced on equipment which processes dairy.

Kosher Gelatin is gelatin from a non-mammal source, usually fish.

Lacto Vegetarian is a vegetarian who eats dairy products but not eggs.

Ovo-Lacto is a vegetarian who does not eat any animals, but does eat eggs and dairy products.

Ovo Vegetarian is a vegetarian who eats eggs but not dairy products.

Pareve (or Parve) symbol (P) indicates that the product does not contain meat or dairy, but may contain fish or eggs.

Vegan is a vegetarian who does not eat any animal products, including honey.

Vegetarian is a person who chooses not to eat some or all animal products.

MILK TERMS[1]

Homogenized milk is a process that breaks up the fat globules (liposomes) in the cream of raw milk by a factor of ten times or more so that the fat molecules become evenly dispersed, rather than separating and floating to the top as occurs in raw milk. Homogenization releases a protein called xanthine oxidase (XO) from the fat globules; XO damages the arteries and is implicated in arteriosclerosis.

Pasteurization involves the heating of a liquid to a specific temperature for a specific amount of time to kill some (not all) bacteria. This process destroys many enzymes that make milk easy to digest, vitamins, proteins, and minerals, and it kills beneficial bacteria (needed to help prevent people from developing allergies to foods.) Milk can be pasteurized by heating to 163 degrees F for fifteen minutes or 145 degrees F for a half-hour.

Skimming milk is a process that reduces milk's fat content, but it also affects our digestion; it allows milk to pass through the stomach quickly and be absorbed before it is fully digested. This is believed to be a major contributor to inflammatory conditions such as arthritis, allergies, skin problems, etc.

Ultra High Temperature Pasteurization involves completely sterilizing the product by raising the temperature to about 285 degrees F for one to two seconds.

"HEALTH" TERMS

Certified Organic means the food has been inspected by a third-party agency to verify organic authenticity to the consumer. Several certification agencies exist. You will see the certification seal or name of the certification agency on the food label. When you see this claim, it means:

- No harmful chemicals have been applied for at least three years.
- The farmer and processor have annual certification inspections.
- They have kept detailed records of their practices.
- They use ecologically-friendly methods and substances to improve the soil and control pests.

Genetic Engineering or GMO is a laboratory technique used to change the DNA of living organisms.

Organic refers to an "earth friendly" method of processing and farming. Organic farmers do not use chemicals in an environmentally harmful manner. Organic agriculture practices cannot ensure that products are completely free of residues. In raising organic animals, hormones and antibiotics may not be used, and the cows are fed only organic feed. Products may still have GMO ingredients.

POWER FOOD TERMS

Antioxidants are a group of vitamins, minerals, and enzymes that help protect our bodies from the formation of free radicals (atoms that cause damage to our cells).

Phytochemicals are non-nutrient plant chemicals that contain protective, disease-preventive compounds. Some phytochemicals include:

- Carotenoids are a group of natural fat-soluble pigments responsible for many of the red, orange, and yellow colors of plant leaves, fruits, and flowers, as well as the colors of some birds, insects, fish, and crustaceans.

Beta carotene and alpha carotene are responsible for the orange color of carrots, and lycopene for the red color of tomatoes. Carotenoids act as antioxidants, protecting cells and tissues from the damaging effects of free radicals.

- *Polyphenols* are a class of phytochemicals found in high concentrations in foods such as grapes.

- *Flavanoids* (Vitamin P) are a class of polyphenols. They are antioxidant molecules found in plant sources such as fruits, flowers, roots, stems, tea, grains, and vegetables. They are often responsible for the coloring of plants. A good rule of nutrition is the more depth of color, the more nutritional content of the fruit or vegetable. Flavanoids enhance the activity of Vitamin C.

There are over four-thousand known flavanoids; they include:

- *Lignans* are a phytochemical found in nuts, whole grains, and cereals. Several lignans, such as secoisolariciresinol, are considered to be phytoestrogens, plant chemicals that mimic the hormone estrogen. These are especially abundant in flaxseed. Bacteria in our intestines convert them into two other lignans, enterolactone and enterodiol, which also have estrogen-like effects.

- *Isoflavones* (genistein, diadzein, glycitein) are a class of flavanoids found in soy that function as antioxidants and possess phytoestrogenic properties.

- *Proanthocyanins* is a polyphenol found in grapes.

- Catechins are polyphenols found in tea, grapes, and cocoa.

- Proanthocyanidins/Tannins are large polyphenol molecules found in tea and nuts.

- Quercetin is an antioxidant and phytoestrogen. It is found in onions, apples, and green tea, and in smaller amounts in beans and vegetables.

- Naringenin has been shown to exhibit anti-estrogenic, antioxidant, and cholesterol lowering activities. It is one of the most abundant polyphenols in tomatoes. It's also found in citrus fruits.

FOOD LABEL TERMS FROM THE US FDA[1]

Free means a product contains no amount of, small or "physiologically inconsequential" amounts of, one or more of: fat, saturated fat, cholesterol, sodium, sugars, and calories. For example, "calorie-free" means fewer than five calories per serving, and "sugar-free" and "fat-free" both mean less than 0.5 g per serving. Synonyms for "free" include "without," "no" and "zero." A synonym for fat-free milk is "skim."

Low can be used on foods that can be eaten frequently without exceeding dietary guidelines for one or more of these components: fat, saturated fat, cholesterol, sodium, and calories. Thus, descriptors are defined as follows:

Low fat contains 3 g or less per serving.

Low saturated fat contains 1 g or less per serving.

Low sodium contains 140 mg or less per serving.

Very low sodium means 35 mg or less per serving.

Low cholesterol has to have 20 mg or less and 2 g or less of saturated fat per serving.

Low-calorie foods contain 40 calories or less per serving.

Synonyms for low include "little," "few," "low source of," and "contains a small amount of."

Lean and extra lean can be used to describe the fat content of meat, poultry, seafood, and game meats.

Lean is less than 10 g fat, 4.5 g or less saturated fat, and less than 95 mg cholesterol per serving and per 100 g.

Extra lean is less than 5 g fat, less than 2 g saturated fat, and less than 95 mg cholesterol per serving and per 100 g.

High can be used if the food contains 20 percent or more of the Daily Value for a particular nutrient in a serving.

Good source means that one serving of a food contains 10 to 19 percent of the Daily Value for a particular nutrient.

Reduced is defined as a nutritionally altered product containing at least 25 percent less of a nutrient or of calories than the regular, or reference, product. However, a reduced claim can't be made on a product if its reference food already meets the requirement for a "low" claim.

Less means that a food, whether altered or not, contains 25 percent less of a nutrient or of calories than the reference food. For example, pretzels that have 25 percent less fat than potato chips could carry a "less" claim. "Fewer" is an acceptable synonym.

Light can mean two things:

First, that a nutritionally altered product contains one-third fewer calories or half the fat of the reference food. If the food derives 50 percent or more of its calories from fat, the reduction must be 50 percent of the fat.

Second, that the sodium content of a low-calorie, low-fat food has been reduced by 50 percent. In addition, "light in sodium" may be used on food in which the sodium content has been reduced by at least 50 percent.

The term "light" still can be used to describe properties such as texture and color, as long as the label explains the intent. (For example, "light brown sugar" and "light and fluffy.")

More means that a serving of food, whether altered or not, contains a nutrient that is at least 10 percent of the Daily Value more than the reference food. The 10 percent of Daily Value also applies to "fortified," "enriched," "added," "extra," and "plus" claims; but in those cases, the food must be altered. but in those cases, the food must be altered.

Alternative spellings of these descriptive terms and their synonyms is allowed—such as "hi" and "lo"—as long as the alternatives are not misleading.

Healthy food must be low in fat and saturated fat and contain limited amounts of cholesterol and sodium. In addition, if it's a single-item food, it must provide at least 10 percent of one or more of vitamins A or C, iron, calcium, protein, or fiber. Exempt from this "10-percent" rule are certain raw, canned, and frozen fruits and vegetables, and certain cereal-grain products. These foods can be labeled "healthy," if they do not contain ingredients that change the nutritional profile, and, in the case of enriched grain products, conform to standards of identity, which call for certain required ingredients. If it's a meal-type product, such as frozen entrees and dinners, it must provide 10 percent of two or three of these vitamins or minerals, or protein or fiber, in addition to meeting the other criteria. The sodium content cannot exceed 360 mg per serving for individual foods and 480 mg per serving for meal-type products.

Percent fat free must be a low-fat or a fat-free product. In addition, the claim must accurately reflect the amount of fat present in 100 g of the food. Thus, if a food contains 2.5 g fat per 50 g, the claim must be "95 percent fat free."

Implied claims are prohibited when they wrongfully imply that a food contains or does not contain a meaningful level of a nutrient. For example, a product claiming to be made with an ingredient known to be a source of fiber (such as "made with oat bran") is not allowed unless the product contains enough of that ingredient (for example, oat bran) to meet the definition for "good source" of fiber. Another example: a claim that a product contains "no tropical oils" is allowed, but only on foods that are "low" in saturated fat because consumers have come to equate tropical oils with high saturated fat.

Meals and main dishes—claims that a meal or main dish is "free" of a nutrient, such as sodium or cholesterol, and must meet the same requirements as those for individual foods. Other claims can be used under special circumstances. For example, "low-calorie" means the meal or main dish contains 120 calories or fewer per 100 g. "Low-sodium" means the food has 140 mg or fewer per 100 g. "Low-cholesterol" means the food contains 20 mg cholesterol or fewer per 100 g and no more than 2 g saturated fat. "Light" means the meal or main dish is low-fat or low-calorie.

Standardized foods are for any nutrient content claim, such as, "reduced fat," "low calorie," and "light." They may be used in conjunction with a standardized term if the new product has been specifically formulated to meet FDA's criteria for that claim, if the product is not nutritionally inferior to the traditional standardized food, and if the new product complies with certain compositional requirements set by FDA. A new product bearing a claim also must have performance characteristics similar to the referenced traditional standardized food. If the product doesn't, and the differences materially limit the product's use, its label must state the differences (for example, not recommended for baking) to inform consumers.

The FDA regulation defines the term "fresh" when it is used to suggest that a food is raw or unprocessed. In this context, "fresh" can be used only on a food that is raw, has never been frozen or heated, and contains no preservatives. (Irradiation at low levels is allowed.) "Fresh frozen," "frozen fresh," and "freshly frozen" can be used for foods that are quickly frozen while still fresh. Blanching (brief scalding before freezing to prevent nutrient breakdown) is allowed.

Other uses of the term "fresh," such as in "fresh milk" or "freshly baked bread," are not affected.

HEALTH CLAIMS FROM THE US FDA[1]

Up to ten relationship claims between a nutrient or a food and the risk of a disease or health-related condition are now allowed. They can be made in several ways: through third-party references (such as the National Cancer Institute), statements, symbols (such as a heart), and vignettes or descriptions. The claim must meet the requirements for authorized health claims; for example, they cannot state the degree of risk reduction and can only use "may" or "might" in discussing the nutrient or food-disease relationship, and they must state that other factors play a role in that disease. The allowed nutrient-disease relationship claims and rules for their use are:

Calcium and osteoporosis claim may be used if a food contains 20 percent or more of the Daily Value for calcium

(200 mg) per serving, has a calcium content that equals or exceeds the food's content of phosphorus, and contains a form of calcium that can be readily absorbed and used by the body. The claim must name the target group most in need of adequate calcium intake (teens and young adult, white and Asian women) and state the need for exercise and a healthy diet. A product that contains 40 percent or more of the Daily Value for calcium must state on the label that a total dietary intake greater than 200 percent of the Daily Value for calcium (2,000 mg or more) has no further known benefit.

Saturated fat and cholesterol, and coronary heart disease (CHD) claim may be used if the food meets the definitions for the nutrient content claim "low saturated fat," "low cholesterol," and "low fat," or, if fish and game meats, for "extra lean." It may mention the link between reduced risk of CHD and lower saturated fat and cholesterol intakes to lower blood cholesterol levels.

Fiber-containing grain products, fruits and vegetables, and cancer claim may be used if a food contains a grain product, fruit or vegetable, and meets the nutrient content claim requirements for "low-fat," and, without fortification, be a "good source" of dietary fiber.

Fruits, vegetables, and grain products that contain fiber, and risk of CHD claim may be used if a food contains fruits, vegetables, and grain products. It also must meet the nutrient content claim requirements for "low saturated fat," "low cholesterol," and "low fat" and contain, without fortification, at least 0.6 g soluble fiber per serving.

Sodium and hypertension (high blood pressure) claim may be used if a food meets the nutrient content claim requirements for "low-sodium."

Fruits and vegetables, and cancer claim may be made for fruits and vegetables that meet the nutrient content claim requirements for "low fat" and that, without fortification, are a "good source" of at least one of the following: dietary fiber or vitamins A or C. This claim relates to diets low in fat and rich in fruits and vegetables (and thus vitamins A and C and dietary fiber) to reduce cancer risk. The FDA authorized this claim in place of an antioxidant vitamin and cancer claim.

Fat and cancer claim indicates that a food meets the nutrient content claim requirements for "low fat" or, if fish and game meats, for "extra lean."

Folic acid and neural tube defects claim is allowed on dietary supplements that contain sufficient folate, and on conventional foods that are naturally good sources of folate, as long as they do not provide more than 100 percent of the Daily Value for vitamin A as retinol or preformed vitamin A or vitamin D. A sample claim is "healthful diets with adequate folate may reduce a woman's risk of having a child with a brain or spinal cord defect."

Dietary sugar alcohols and dental caries (cavities) claim applies to food products, such as candy or gum, containing the sugar alcohols xylitol, sorbitol, mannitol, malitol, isomalt, lactitol, hydrogenated starch hydrolysates, hydrogenated glucose syrups, or a combination. If the food also contains a fermentable carbohydrate, such as sugar, the food cannot lower the pH of plaque in the mouth below 5.7. In addition to the food ingredients' relationship to dental caries, the claim also must state that frequent between-meal consumption of foods high in sugars and starches promotes tooth decay. A shortened claim is allowed on food packages with less than fifteen square inches of labeling.

Soluble fiber from certain foods, such as whole oats and psyllium seed husk, and heart disease claim must state that the fiber also needs to be part of a diet low in saturated fat and cholesterol, and the food must provide sufficient soluble fiber. The amount of soluble fiber in a serving of the food must be listed on the Nutrition Facts panel.

INGREDIENT LABELING[1]

Under NLEA (the Nutrition Labeling and Education Act), some foods are exempt from nutrition labeling. These include:

- Food served for immediate consumption, such as that served in hospital cafeterias and airplanes, and that sold by food service vendors; for example, mall cookie counters, sidewalk vendors, and vending machines.

- Ready-to-eat food that is not for immediate consumption but is prepared primarily on site; for example, bakery, deli, and candy store items.

- Food shipped in bulk, as long as it is not for sale in that form to consumers.

- Medicinal foods, such as those used to address the nutritional needs of patients with certain diseases.

- Plain coffee and tea, some spices, and other foods that contain no significant amounts of nutrients.

Ingredient declaration is required on all foods that have more than one ingredient.

Because people may be allergic to certain additives and

to help them better avoid them, the ingredient list must include, when appropriate:

- FDA-certified color additives, such as FD&C Blue No. 1, by name.

- Sources of protein hydrolysates, which are used in many foods as flavors and flavor enhancers.

- Declaration of caseinate as a milk derivative in the ingredient list of foods that claim to be non-dairy, such as coffee whiteners.

As required by NLEA, beverages that claim to contain juice must declare the total percentage of juice on the information panel. In addition, FDA's regulation establishes criteria for naming juice beverages. For example, when the label of a multi-juice beverage states one or more—but not all—of the juices present, and the predominantly named juice is present in minor amounts, the product's name must state that the beverage is flavored with that juice or declare the amount of the juice in a 5 percent range; for example, "raspberry-flavored juice blend" or "juice blend, 2 to 7 percent raspberry juice."

DAILY VALUES—DRVs[1]

The new label reference value, "Daily Value," comprises two sets of dietary standards: Daily Reference Values (DRVs) and Reference Daily Intakes (RDIs). To make label reading less confusing (they didn't do a very good job!), only the Daily Value term appears on the label.

DRVs have been established for macronutrients that are sources of energy: fat, saturated fat, total carbohydrate (including fiber), and protein; and for cholesterol, sodium and potassium, which do not contribute calories.

DRVs for the energy-producing nutrients are based on the number of calories consumed per day. A daily intake of 2,000 calories has been established as the reference. This level was chosen, in part, because it approximates the caloric requirements for postmenopausal women. This group has the highest risk for excessive intake of calories and fat.

DRVs for the energy-producing nutrients are calculated as follows:

- Fat based on 30 percent of calories

- Saturated fat based on 10 percent of calories

- Carbohydrate based on 60 percent of calories

- Protein based on 10 percent of calories (The DRV for protein applies only to adults and children over four. RDIs for protein for special groups have been established.)

- Fiber based on 11.5 g of fiber per 1,000 calories

Because of current public health recommendations, DRVs for some nutrients represent the **uppermost** limit (which you should never reach!) that is considered desirable. The DRVs for total fat, saturated fat, cholesterol, and sodium are:

- Total fat less than 65 g

- Saturated fat less than 20 g

- Cholesterol less than 300 mg

- Sodium less than 2,400 mg

	Fictitious Food Label
Step 1.	**Nutrition Facts** Serving Size 1 Cup (228 g) Servings per container 3
Step 2.	**Amount Per Serving** **Calories 250** Calories from Fat 110

Step 3.	% **Daily Value***
	Total Fat 12 g 18%
	    Saturated Fat 3 g 15%
	    Trans Fat 1.5 g
	Cholesterol 30 mg 10%
	Sodium 470 mg 20%

Step 4.	**Total Carbohydrate** 31 g 10%
	    Dietary Fiber 0 0%
	    Sugars 5g

Step 5.	**Protein** 5 g Vitamin A 4% Vitamin C 2% Calcium 15%
Step 6. % DV	Iron 5%

Percent Daily Values are based on a 2,000 calorie diet. Your daily values may be higher or lower, depending on your calorie needs.

	Calories:	2,000	2,500
Total Fat	Less than	65 g	80 g
Sat. Fat	Less than	20 g	25 g
Cholesterol	Less than	300 mg	300 mg
Sodium	Less than	2400 mg	2400 mg
Total Carbohydrate		300 g	375 mg
Dietary Fiber		25 g	30 mg

DECODING OF A FOOD LABEL

1. To begin, read the serving size and the servings per container. Compare this to how much you actually eat. The size of the serving on the package affects all the nutrient amounts listed on the top part of the label. In the sample label left, one serving equals one cup. If you ate the whole package, you would eat three cups. That triples the calories and other nutrient numbers, including the % Daily Values as shown below. (See Calories and % Daily Value for more information.)

2. Calories provide a measure of how much energy you get from a serving of this food. The label also tells you how many of the calories in one serving come from fat. In the example, there are 250 calories in a serving. How many calories from fat are there in ONE serving? Answer: 110 calories, which means almost half comes from fat. What if you ate the whole package? Then, you would consume three servings, or 750 calories, and 330 would come from fat.

3. Americans generally eat these nutrients in adequate amounts, or even too much. Eating too much fat, saturated fat, trans fat, cholesterol, or sodium may increase your risk of certain chronic diseases, like heart disease, some cancers, or high blood pressure. I recommend keeping your intake of saturated fat and cholesterol low and eating absolutely no trans fat as part of a nutritionally balanced diet.

4. When looking at a food label you may find that it lists high sugar. Check the label to find out the source of

sugar. Try to limit or avoid added sugar—especially "white" sugar! Try to consume whole foods that naturally contain sugar, such as fruit.

5. Americans rarely get enough dietary fiber, vitamin A, vitamin C, calcium, and iron in their diets. Eating enough of these nutrients can improve your health and help reduce the risk of some diseases and conditions (See Nutrition Studies in Appendix). If your diet consists of a variety of whole foods you should not have to worry (See Chapter 5.)

6. For labeling purposes, the FDA set 2,000 calories as the reference amount for calculating % DVs. The % DV shows you the percent (how much) of the recommended daily amount of a nutrient is in a serving of food. By using the % DV, you can tell if this amount is high or low—even if you don't consume 2,000 calories. The FDA considers % DVs under 5 low and over 20 high. Look for products with nutrients over twenty.

NOTES

6

CRACKING THE CODE
OF INGREDIENTS

HAVE YOU EVER looked at the ingredients list on a box of food and said "What is that? I can't even pronounce that word." While ingredients such as corn starch may be familiar to most, ingredients such as butylated hydroxytoluene are not. To confuse you even more (and get your money) manufacturers use different names for the same ingredient!

Remember, even though a food is in the "health food" section does not mean it is healthier.

Don't be confused any longer. Grab your food boxes and get ready to "crack the code"!

VEGETARIAN TERMS

Agar is a gelling agent made from red saltwater algae.

Arrowroot is a fine white starch with thickening properties superior to those of flour and corn starch. Arrowroot can be used for both sauces and desserts.

Brewer's Yeast is a health supplement grown on molasses, sugar beets, or wood pulp. A rich source of vitamin B and protein.

Dulse is a natural sea vegetable rich in proteins and minerals. It has a soft, chewy texture. It can be purchased as leaves, flakes, granules, or powders. It is fat, sugar, and cholesterol free.

Eddamme are soybeans that have been harvested when the beans are still green and sweet. You can boil and eat them for a snack or in your favorite dish.

Essential Fatty Acids (Vitamin F) are fatty acids that cannot be made by the body and must be supplied through the diet. These fatty acids are also known as polyunsaturates, and are recommended for lowering cholesterol and blood pressure and reducing the risk of heart disease. Ideally we need more linolenic, about a 2:1 ratio. (The American ratio is not good—20 [Omega 6]:1 [Omega 3].)

- *Alpha-Linolenic Acid* (Omega 3) flax, marine source of food or supplements

- *Linoleic Acid* (Omega 6) dominant in vegetable oils such as safflower, sunflower, peanut, and corn oils

Flaxseeds are reddish-brown seeds from the flax plant which can be eaten raw or pressed into oil. An excellent source of lignans, fiber, and linolenic acid (most oils contain linoleic too). Current methods of manufacturing polyunsaturated oils have removed much of these important fats from our food chain. Should be stored in refrigerator and eaten raw, as heat destroys the nutrients. Do not fry; baking is OK.

Hummus is a blend of pureed chickpeas, lemon, tahini, oil, and spices.

Miso is a salty condiment used in Japanese cooking. It is a mixture of soybeans, malted rice, and salt.

Rennet is an enzyme from the stomach of calves, used to coagulate cheese. Found in many but not all dairy cheeses. Vegetarian foods will sometimes use a vegetable rennet derived from plants instead.

Soy (Soybean) is an Asian legume and the only plant source of protein considered a complete protein. Look for non-GMO (not genetically modified) and organic soy products.

Soy Protein ingredients are made from soybeans which are processed into flakes. Defatted soy flakes are the basis for making the three primary soy protein ingredients:

1. *Soy Flour* is made from ground roasted soybeans. It contains 40 (full fat)-50 (defatted) percent protein. It comes in full fat, defatted, and lecithinated. Full fat contains the natural oils found in soybean; defatted removes the fat in processing; lecithinated has lecithin added during processing. Soy flour is the least refined of the three sources.

2. *Soy Protein Concentrate* is made from defatted soy flakes by removing (with alcohol or water) most of the sugar. It contains most of the fiber and about 70 percent protein on a dry weight basis. It is lower in carbohydrates than soy flour. Using alcohol in

processing removes valuable phytochemicals; water washing retains most of the valuable phytochemicals. Processing methods are important.

3. *Isolated Soy Protein or Soy Protein Isolate* is a refined product made when protein is removed from defatted soy flakes. It contains about 92 percent protein on a dry weight basis, with nearly all the fat and carbohydrates removed.

Tahini is a smooth, rich paste made from ground sesame seeds.

Tempeh is a vegetarian replacement for meat, made from fermented soybeans. Originally from Indonesia.

Textured Soy Protein / Textured Vegetable Protein is a popular but highly refined vegetarian replacement for meat. It is made from textured soy flour and textured soy protein concentrates. It may cause gastric distress.

Textured Soy Flour is made by running defatted soy flour into a cooker. It contains about 50 percent protein, fiber, and soluble fiber. It is used as a meat extender.

Textured Soy Protein Concentrate is made from extrusion. It contains about 70 percent protein and fiber.

Tofu is a vegetarian replacement for meat, eggs, and cheese made from curdled soy milk pressed into blocks. Tofu can be eaten fresh or cooked in many different ways and is an excellent source of protein. Originally from China.

1. Extra-Firm Tofu—frying, roasting, grilling, and marinating

2. Firm Tofu (Chinese-style)—stir-frying, boiling, filling

3. Soft Tofu (Japanese-style)—puréeing

4. Silken Tofu (smooth, custard-like)—puréeing, simmering, egg substitution

GRAIN TERMS

Amaranth is a protein-rich seed that is commonly used as a cereal grain.

Barley is an ancient, hardy grain. Barley contains five parts. The two outer parts are protective hulls which cannot be eaten. Inside the hull is the aleurone, which protects the endosperm. The endosperm contains most of the starch in the grain. The center is the pearl. (This is where "pearled" barley comes from.)

Basmati is a creamy textured long-grain rice. It can be polished (white) or whole-grain (brown).

Buckwheat is a seed often prepared like rice. The crushed, hulled kernels are often used for dishes such as kasha.

Bulgur Wheat is a quick cooking form of whole wheat that has been cleaned, parboiled, dried, and crushed and has a variety of textures. It is used in many grain-based dishes.

Brown Rice is the whole grain of rice with only the (inedible) outer layer husk removed. Brown rice can be long-, medium-, or short-grain.

Fiber is a complex carbohydrate that is not digestible and does not absorb into your bloodstream. It is not a nutrient nor does it give the body energy. It does promote health in many ways. There are two types of fiber:

1. *Soluble Fiber,* such as oat bran, dissolves in water. It is often used in low-fat and non-fat foods to add texture and consistency. Fibers called gums, mucilages, and

pectin are all soluble. Soluble fiber such as pectin binds to fatty substances in your body and promotes their excretion as waste. This seems to help lower cholesterol levels. Soluble fibers also help regulate the body's use of sugars.

2. *Insoluble Fiber,* the "roughage that sweeps the colon," gives structure to plant walls. This group is known as cellulose, hemicellulose, and lignan. Wheat bran is high in insoluble fiber.

Gliadin is a protein obtained by alcoholic extraction of gluten from wheat and rye.

Hominy is the dried corn kernel with the hull removed. It is usually soaked in liquid, cooled, and used in stews or casseroles. Corn is actually a whole grain.

Kamut is not a grain but a brand name. Kamut brand grain is a relative of durum (also known as duram or durham) wheat. It has a buttery flavor and contains more protein and nutrients than common wheat.

Millet is a small, round, yellow grain. It is a bland grain that is used for mixed dishes, cereals, flour, and bread.

Rye is a dark cereal grain that adds flavor to many foods. Most rye that is used in such items as breads is not full grain rye but a combination of rye and processed wheat.

Spelt is one of the original grains mentioned in the Bible. It has a higher water solubility, so the nutrients are easily absorbed by the body. It is full of fiber, nutrients, and has more protein than common wheat.

Triticale is a modern grain developed of rye and wheat. It has a nutty flavor with more protein and less gluten than wheat alone. It is used in grain-based dishes and foods.

Quinoa is a small, ivory, bead-shaped grain that cooks like rice—but faster. It is higher in protein than other grains, and is a good source of iron and magnesium. Quinoa can be used in many dishes that call for rice.

Wheat Berries are whole grains that haven't been processed. They are usually cooked and used in grain-based dishes. Cracked wheat is wheat berries that have been crushed. You can also purchase *Rye Berries*.

Wheat Gluten, also known as seitan, is a wheat protein that has a chewy, meaty texture. Wheat, rye, oats, barley, and buckwheat all contain gluten.

Whole Grain is the edible part of any grain (wheat, corn, oats, and rice) It contains:

- *Endosperm* is the inner part of the grain. It contains the most protein and carbohydrates. White flour is ground from the endosperm (no bran or germ).

- *Bran* is the outer layers of the grain. It supplies large amounts of B-vitamins, trace minerals, and dietary fiber.

- *Germ* is a small but important part of the bran. It sprouts, generating a new plant. It has B-vitamins, trace minerals, and some protein.

Wild Rice is the seed of a water grass. It has a nut-like flavor, and is often used in place of (or mixed with) grains. Because it's a seed it is high in protein.

MILK TERMS

Lactose is a milk sugar made up of glucose and galactose. Galactose has been identified as a factor in heart disease and cataracts. Most adults do not have the enzyme to break down lactose. Instead, lactose is broken down by bacteria in the lower intestines causing their own body wastes to combine with the sugars and ferment into gas and toxins, causing bloating and cramps.

Whey Protein is what is left after fat and casein are removed from the milk.

Curd is the part of the milk that coagulates when the milk sours or is treated with enzymes.

FOOD ADDITIVE TERMS

Food additives are substances added to foods to perform specific functions. These include:

1. Preserving the food (to increase the shelf life or slow the growth of microorganisms)

2. Changing the appearance or taste of the food (by adding color or flavor)

3. Processing the food (by adding special agents that help the ingredients stay together).

Additives such as salt, vegetable food colorings, and honey have been used for centuries. Additives may be natural or artificial.

Natural additives are substances found naturally in a food and are extracted to be used in another. For example, beetroot juice with its bright purple color can be used to color other foods such as sweets.

Artificial additives can be:

1. Substances made *synthetically*. That is, they are not natural. An example is azodicarbonamide, a flour

improver that is used to help bread dough hold together.

2. *Nature Identical*—Substances that are man-made copies of substances that are found in nature. For example, benzoic acid is a natural substance but it can also be made synthetically and used as a preservative.

Additives are used to:

- keep food fresh until it is eaten
- make food look or taste better
- ensure that the food is convenient to store or use
- keep the price of food competitive
- make food healthier (higher in vitamins or lower in fat)
- aid in processing and manufacturing

Acids and Alkalis are used to neutralize the acidity or alkalinity of certain foods. Citric acid is an example.

Antioxidants delay the process of oxidation in unsaturated fats and oils, colorings, and flavorings. Oxidation is caused when the fats in the food combine with oxygen and turn food rancid. Rancid fats lead to flavor and color changes, taste unpleasant, and are a health risk. Antioxidants are also used in fruits, vegetables, and juices to extend the shelf life.

Carcinogen is a chemical or other agent that causes cancer in animals or humans.

Chelating Agents trap small amounts of metal atoms that would otherwise cause food to discolor or go rancid.

Colors are used to make food look more pleasing. During processing, color can be lost, so additives are used to restore the original color. Color additives are also used to make existing color brighter. Most colors are either natural or nature identical and some colors are also vitamins; these are the only colors allowed in baby foods.

Emulsifiers and Stabilizers: Stabilizers mix together ingredients like oil and water that would normally separate; stabilizers prevent the mixture from separating again. They are used in foods such as ice cream. Lecithin, gelatin, and pectin are commonly used natural emulsifiers.

Flavor Enhancers are used to accentuate the natural flavor of foods. They are most often used when very little of a natural ingredient is present. Monosodium glutamate (MSG) is an example of a flavor enhancer.

Preservatives help keep food safe longer, which gives consumers the ability to buy foods in advance of using them so they do not have to shop as often. Preservatives also give stores the ability to offer a wider selection of foods, as foods can be safely imported or made available out of season.

Sweeteners are either Intense or Bulk. Intense sweeteners (saccharin and aspartame) are many times sweeter than sugar and so are only used in tiny amounts. This makes them suitable for use in products such as diet drinks, which are very low in energy. Bulk sweeteners (such as sorbitol) have a similar sweetness to sugar so are used in similar amounts.

Thickening Agents are natural or chemically modified carbohydrates that absorb some water present in food, making the food thicker. Thickening agents "stabilize" factory-made foods by keeping the complex mixtures of oils, water, acids, and solids well mixed. Propylene glycol is an example of a thickening agent.

COMMON "HEALTH FOOD" ADDITIVES: SOME GOOD...SOME NOT SO GOOD!

Listed below are some common food additives found in health foods. Your best bet is to eat whole foods with no additives, preservatives, or modifications all or most of the time.

Alginate is a derivative of seaweed (kelp). It is used as a thickening agent for ice cream, cheese, candy, and yogurt.

Alpha Tocopherol (Vitamin E) is an additive abundant in whole wheat, rice germ, and vegetable oils. It is destroyed by the refining and bleaching of flour. It prevents oils from going rancid. Studies indicate that large amounts of vitamin E may help reduce the risk of heart disease and cancer.

Ascorbic Acid/Sodium Ascorbate/Erythorbic Acid is vitamin C. It can also be synthetic.

Beta Carotene is an antioxidant used as a coloring and to add nutrient to a food.

Carageenan is a thickening and stabilizing agent obtained from seaweed. It is used in ice cream, jelly, chocolate milk, and infant formula.

Casein/Sodium Caseinate is the principal protein in milk. It is used as a thickening and whitening agent. It is used in ice cream, ice milk, sherbet, coffee creamers, and a lot of "non-dairy" and "vegetarian" foods.

Citric Acid is abundant naturally in citrus fruits and berries. It is used as a strong acid, tart flavoring, and antioxidant. It is also used as a thickening and chelating agent in foods such as ice cream, sherbet, fruit drinks, candy, carbonated beverages, and instant potatoes.

Cellulose is the main element of the fiber of plants. It is used as a thickener and stabilizer.

Gluten (wheat and corn) is the principal protein component in cereal grains. It is used in dough (wheat); to extend the protein of a food (corn); and to improve the texture in baked goods (vital wheat gluten).

Glycerin forms the backbone of fat and oil molecules. It maintains water content and is used for candy, fudge, baked goods, etc.

Glucose is found in many fruits, vegetables, and grains but also occurs in animal sources.

Gums (arabic, cellulose, guar, locust bean, xanthan, etc., are obtained from natural sources—bushes, trees, seaweed, etc.) They are used as a thickening agent and stabilizer in foods such as pudding, dough, cottage cheese, and ice cream.

Gypsum is a naturally occurring calcium sulfate used as a coagulant to make tofu.

Magnesium Salts such as magnesium chloride are used for a variety of purposes such as binders, firming agents, flavor enhancers, etc. Magnesium is an essential nutrient needed in human diets.

Monoglycerides and Diglycerides are fats produced from natural vegetable sources such as soybean, cottonseed, palm, or sunflower and mixed with glycerin. They are used as emulsifiers to prevent separation and are sodium free.

Nagari is a naturally occurring coagulant (binding/thickening agent) containing mostly magnesium chloride and other minerals found in sea water (except sodium chloride).

Natural Colors such as paprika, turmeric, and saffron are used in such things as soy cheese to change the color.

Oligofructose is produced from chicory roots. It is not absorbed in the small intestine, but is partly digested in the large intestine. It has a slightly sweet taste and provides less than about half as many calories per gram as fructose or other sugar. It is used as a bulking agent, emulsifier, and prebiotic. (It promotes the growth of "good" bifidus bacteria).

Phosphates are the drug form (salt) of phosphorus. Phosphates naturally occur in our food, our bodies, and in water. They are formed when some or all of the hydrogen of a phosphoric acid is replaced with metals. Excess quantities may lead to dietary imbalances and thus health problems.

Salt is a refined product with all the minerals removed and usually contains other ingredients such as sugar (dextrose), aluminum, and iodide.

Sea Salt is derived from the sea. Due to high demand, several manufacturers process this salt the same as refined table salt. Look for unrefined, sun-dried sea salt with nothing added.

Starch is a white granular organic chemical produced by all green plants such as potato, tapioca, corn, wheat, rice.

Modified Starch refers to a chemical modification such as bleaching and oxidation. (Do not use.) Unmodified starch is just that—unmodified; this is what you should look for in health foods.

Vegetable Oil Sterols are substances extracted from soybeans that reduce the absorption of cholesterol from food and lower blood cholesterol levels. They may reduce the body's absorption of carotenoids.

SUGARS YOU WILL FIND IN "HEALTH FOOD"

(See Appendix 4 for sugar facts.)

Agave is derived from the blue agave plant. It is absorbed more slowly than common sugar and contains nutrients.

Amasake is a sweetener made from sweet brown rice.

Barley Malt Syrup is made from soaked, sprouted, or dried barley. It is about 40 percent complex carbohydrates and 3 percent protein. Rye and wheat malts are also available but are less common.

Carob tastes similar to chocolate but does not contain caffeine or additives. It is about 46 percent natural sugars. It also contains some protein, B vitamins, and potassium.

Date Sugar is made of dehydrated ground dates. It contains fructose, sucrose, glucose, and all the nutrients found in dates.

Evaporated Cane Juice/Dried Cane Juice/Cane Juice/ Naturally Milled Sugar/Unrefined Cane Sugar is processed by a single-step rather than a multiple-step crystallization process, therefore retaining more of the character of the juice from which it is recovered. Sugar cane is cut not burned. It is processed mechanically rather than with chemicals. Sugar cane syrup is spun to remove molasses, then dried and packaged. Although healthier, it is still a refined product (and the most commonly used in "health foods").

Fruit Juice Concentrates are usually derived from apples, grapes, peaches, pears, and pineapple. They are mainly fructose and sucrose. Commercial fruit juices or concentrates may contain a high amount of pesticides.

Fruit Sugar is fructose and gluctose. Fructose (chemically named levulose) is found in fruits and honey.

Maltose is malt sugar found in amasake, barley, and rice syrup. It is a disaccharide, thus metabolizes slower.

Molasses from the first boil is the finest grade due to the small amount of sugar removed. The second boil takes on a darker color, is less sweet, and has a more pronounced flavor. It is about 50-70 percent sucrose. There are three major types of molasses:

1. *Sulphured Molasses* is made from green sugar cane and is treated with sulphur fumes during the extraction process.

2. *Unsulphured* is the best quality. It is made from the juice of sun-ripened cane and the juice is clarified and concentrated. If you choose molasses make sure it's unsulphured molasses.

3. *Blackstrap* is made from the third boil and used most often in cattle feed. It contains more nutrients than lighter varieties.

Pure Maple Syrup is made from the sap of the northern sugar maple trees. If it is not labeled "Pure Maple Syrup" it may be made with corn syrup (about 65 percent sucrose).

Rapadura sugar is the dried whole natural juice of cane sugar. It is never separated from the molasses; therefore, it retains all the vitamins and minerals available from sugar cane.

Raw Honey is made from the stomach of bees. It is not pasteurized and is unfiltered. It is rich in sucrose so absorbs quickly, but because of its sweetness you can use less. It contains valuable vitamins, minerals, and enzymes. It is nature-made by bees and is a great whole food sweetener.

Types include (depending on where the bees buzz): buckwheat, alfalfa, avocado, clover, eucalyptus, orange blossom, tupelo.

Raw Sugar is white table sugar just before the molasses is extracted. It contains 96 percent sucrose and a trace amount of minerals.

Rice Syrup is often made from cooked rice and sprouted barley. It has the highest protein content of all the sweeteners and contains some B vitamins and potassium (especially when made from brown rice). It contains maltose, glucose, and complex carbohydrates. It is used in baked goods. Use brown rice syrup in cookies, crisps, granola, pies and puddings.

Stevia is a shrub from South Africa. The leaf is used as a sweetener. It is 100 to 300 times sweeter than sugar, but provides no calories. Animal tests and the extensive Japanese experience with stevia suggest that this is a safe herb. Evidence from most studies suggests that stevia is not a concern at *normal* doses. Safety in young children, pregnant or nursing women, or those with severe liver or kidney disease has not been conclusively established. There have not been enough U.S. studies for the FDA to approve stevia as a sugar substitute.

Sorbic Acid/Potassium Sorbate occurs naturally in many plants. It is used as a preservative to prevent mold in cheese, syrup, dried fruits, etc.

Sorghum is the concentrated juice of a plant called sweet sorghum. It's about 65 percent sucrose with some minerals.

Sucanat used to be processed like rapadura but is now being processed like dehydrated cane juice.

Turbinado Sugar is sugar cane or sugar beets at a stage

between raw and refined sugar. It is about 95 percent sucrose.

COMMON ADDITIVES AND PRESERVATIVES TO AVOID

Caffeine is a naturally occurring stimulant in coffee, cocoa, and added to sodas. It is a drug, and because it increases the risks of miscarriages and possible birth defects, inhibits fetal growth, causes headaches, withdrawal symptoms, and a host of other problems, you should avoid caffeine or limit it to small quantities (decaffeinated).

Calcium Propionate (Sodium Propionate) is a calcium salt used to prevent mold growth on bread and rolls.

Calcium Sorbate is a synthetic preservative.

EDTA (ethylenediaminetetraacetic acid) is a chelating agent used in foods such as salad dressing, margarine, sandwich spreads, mayonnaise, processed fruits and vegetables, canned shellfish, and soft drinks. EDTA traps metals (found in food from soil, machinery, and processing) that would otherwise cause rancidity and the breakdown of artificial colors.

*Food Coloring*s such as Blue 1, Blue 2, Citrus Red 2, Red 40, Yellow 6, etc., are man-made colors. Studies of some suggest they caused brain tumors in rats; for others, allergic reactions. Like other often accepted chemicals, many are eventually banned due to the severe problems they caused (such as cancer).

MSG (Monosodium Glutamate) is an amino acid used as a flavor enhancer. It can cause many problems from headaches to breathing difficulties.

Nitrates and Nitrites are used in cured meats such as hot dogs and bacon. They can lead to the formation of cancer-causing chemicals, particularly in bacon. Several studies have linked the consumption—even by children—to cancer.

Propylene Glycol Alginate is a chemically modified algine, thickens acidic foods such as soda pop and salad dressing. It also can stabilize the foam in beer.

Sulfites (Sulfur Dioxide, Sodium Bisulfite) are preservatives used to prevent discoloration. They destroy vitamin B-1 and cause severe reactions—even death.

SYNTHETIC ANTIOXIDANTS TO AVOID

BHA (Butylated Hydroxyanisole) is a synthetic antioxidant used in cereals, chewing gum, potato chips, and vegetable oil. Studies have shown it to cause cancer in rats.

BHT (Butylated Hydroxytoluene) is a synthetic antioxidant used in cereals, chewing gum, etc. It has been shown to increase cancer in animal studies. Residues of BHT occur in human fat.

Propyl gallate is a synthetic antioxidant. It can cause stomach and skin irritation.

STABILIZERS, EMULSIFIERS, & FLAVOR ENHANCERS

Albumin is from animals' blood and is found in dairy and eggs. It is used as a thickener and coagulant.

Brominated Vegetable Oil (BVO) is an emulsifier and clouding agent used in soft drinks. It keeps flavor in oils in suspension and gives a cloudy appearance to citrus-flavored soft drinks. Eating BVO leaves residues in body fat.

COMMON SWEETENERS

Acesulfame-K (the K is the chemical symbol for potassium) is an artificial sweetener sold as Sweet One and Sunett. It is used in baked goods, chewing gum, gelatin desserts, soft drinks, diet drinks, and shakes. The Center for Science in the Public Interest (CSPI) warns "Everyone should avoid this." It is unsafe.

Aspartame is an artificial sweetener used in foods such as diet foods, soft drinks, gelatin, and desserts. It has caused dizziness, hallucinations, headaches, and behavioral problems and may be a carcinogen.

Brown Sugar is refined white sugar with molasses added to it. It promotes tooth decay and is used in highly processed foods.

Corn Syrup is processed by treating corn starch with acids and enzymes. It can also be treated with enzymes to convert some of its dextrose to fructose, which results in high fructose corn syrup. It is used as a sweetener and thickener in foods such as syrups, imitation dairy foods, and candy. Corn syrup promotes tooth decay and is used in highly processed foods.

Cyclamate is an artificial sweetener used in diet foods. Studies indicate that it increases the potency of other carcinogens and may cause harm to the testes.

Dextrose is made of corn, sugar beets, or sugar cane. It is a highly refined monosaccharide and thus quickly absorbed.

Invert Sugar or total invert sugar is part glucose and

fructose. It can also be found naturally in fruits and honey, but it is commonly produced synthetically for commercial use. It is made from the hydrolysis of sucrose.

Mannitol can be derived from plants, most commonly seaweed, but commercial grade mannitol is derived from sugar.

Saccharin is used in dietetic foods or as a tabletop sugar substitute. Many studies on animals have shown it to cause cancer.

Sorbitol is a sweet-tasting sugar alcohol that occurs naturally in berries and fruits, but it is also made industrially from hydrogen and glucose. It can cause gastrointestinal problems ranging from mild discomfort to severe diarrhea with as little as 10-50 gms. It also has been suspected of causing cataracts. Due to their size, children may be affected by smaller amounts.

Sucralose is an artificial sweetener most commonly marketed as Splenda. This synthetic chemical is made by chemically reacting sugar with chlorine.

Sucrose is common table sugar made from cane and sugar beets that has been stripped down and has no nutrients and lots of calories (see "Studies" in Appendices).

Tagatose is a new sugar substitute that is chemically similar to glucose but contains only one-third as many calories. It is poorly absorbed by the body and in large amounts may cause diarrhea, nausea, and gas.

NATURE'S FOOD ADDITIVES

Natural Spices and Herbs such as pepper, onion, garlic, dill, mustard seed.

Vegetable Colorings such as paprika and turmeric.

Thickeners such as seaweed and pectin.

Preservatives such as vitamin E and sea salt.

Natural Sweeteners such as raw honey, fruit, pure maple syrup, rice syrup, malts, unsulphured molasses, amasake, agave and rapadura.*

*Added sugars in foods should be limited. Nature's foods already come with sugar. Read labels.

Let's get back to the basics.

FOODS TO AVOID

Hydrogenated Fats promote cardiovascular disease and obesity.

Artificial Food Colors cause allergies, asthma, hyperactivity, and are a possible carcinogen.

Nitrates and Nitrites can develop into nitrosamines in the body, which can be carcinogenic.

Sulfites can cause allergies and allergic reactions.

Artificial Sweeteners are associated with behavioral problems, hyperactivity, and may be carcinogenic. The government cautions against use of any type of artificial sweetener by children or pregnant women.

MSG causes common allergic and behavioral reactions including headache, dizziness, depression, and mood swings.

Artificial Preservatives such as BHA, BHT, and EDTA may cause allergic reactions, hyperactivity, and cancer.

Artificial Flavors may cause allergic reactions and behavioral problems.

Refined Flour is low in nutrients and is an ingredient of high-processed, high-calorie foods.

Excessive Salt causes fluid retention and increase in blood pressure.

Artificial Fat causes diarrhea and digestive problems.

NOTES

7

THE REAL "DIET" FOODS

WHEN YOU CAN feel good, why feel bad? That's what "power foods" are all about. They are whole foods that contain natural medicinal properties such as antioxidants, vitamins, proteins, phytoestrogens, and bioflavanoids. If you eat a whole foods or mostly whole foods diet you will notice a great difference in your energy, mood, overall health, and productivity. Whole foods are what I suggest you eat all or most of the time. They are minimally processed foods such as vegetables, fruits, beans, and grains. They generally don't have a label or don't need one as they contain one ingredient such as "apple." You can find these anywhere, even your local grocery. When looking for spices look for fresh (whole) or ground. Keep it simple!

To help with your meal planning, this chapter contains lists of whole food items and whole food sources of nutrients.

FRUITS

Apples	Raisins	Cantaloupes
Bananas	Blueberries	Persimmons
Pears	Papayas	Apricots
Prunes	Raspberries	Pomegranates
Peaches	Dates	Figs
Strawberries	Mangos	Ugli fruits
Cherries	Lemons	Cranberries
Kiwis	Oranges	Tangerines
Avocados	Grapes	Grapefruits
Watermelons	Plums	Mangosteens
Guavas	Pineapples	
Starfruits		

VEGETABLES

Broccoli	Arugula	Alfalfa sprouts
Zucchini	Celery	Seaweed
Cauliflower	Mushrooms	Kelp
Peas	Cucumbers	Okra
Asparagus	Tomatoes	Water chestnuts
Cabbage	Barley	Bok choy
Squash	Red peppers	Beets
Garlic	Green peppers	Dakons
Carrots	Pumpkins	Leeks
Fennel	Zucchini	Radishes
Yams	Eggplants	Spirulina
Ginger	Brussel sprouts	Green beans
Spinach	Bamboo shoots	

WHOLE GRAINS AND LEGUMES

May be eaten as flour, whole grain breads, cereal (hot or cold), etc., or in whole form (corn, rice, beans).

Oats (steel-cut)	Arborio	Buckwheat
Brown rice	Bulgur wheat	Barley
Amaranth	Millet	Rye
Sprouted grains	Corn	

LEGUMES (PEAS AND BEANS)

Soybeans	White beans	Split peas
Lima Beans	Lentils	Black beans
Kidney beans	Tempeh	Pinto beans
Garbanzo beans	Navy beans	Tofu
(chickpeas)		

PROTEINS

I recommend a vegetarian diet. Protein sources for vegetarians include whole grains/legumes, nuts, and seeds. If you must eat meat, eat organically raised, chemical-free animals*. Consider meat a luxury food eaten on special occasions.

*The fish listed below have been shown to contain lower levels of mercury. If eating fish, make sure it is tested and shown (read label or contact company) not to contain harmful levels of mercury and other toxins.

WILD GAME   FISH   EGGS

WILD GAME	FISH	EGGS
Deer	Salmon	Organic, free-range
Sheep	Orange roughy	
Goat	Tilapia	
Chicken		
Quail		
Turkey		

FATS AND OILS

SEEDS   NUTS   OILS

SEEDS	NUTS	OILS
Flax	Almonds	Cold-pressed
Sesame	Walnuts	extra virgin olive oil
Sunflower	Hazelnuts	
Pumpkin	Chestnuts	
	Pistachios	
	Brazil nuts	
	Peanuts	
	Pecans	

HERBS AND SPICES

Basil	Marjoram	Rosemary
Thyme	Mint	Saffron
Cumin	Poppy seed	Cayenne
Italian parsley	Pure vanilla	Tarragon
Oregano	Sesame seed	Bay leaf
Paprika	Sage	Mustard seed
Parsley	Black pepper	Cilantro

CONDIMENTS

Raw honey	Apple cider vinegar
Balsamic vinegar	Rice vinegar

WHOLE-FOOD SOURCES OF NUTRIENTS

VITAMIN A (BETA CAROTENE)	VITAMIN B1 (THIAMINE)	VITAMIN B5 (PANTOTHENIC ACID)
Alfalfa	Brewer's Yeast	Beans
Beets	Whole grains	Mother's milk
Carrots	Wheat germ	Fresh vegetables
Garlic	Dried beans	Whole wheat
Papayas	Brown rice	
Sweet potatoes	Soybeans	
Pumpkin	Rice bran	
Apricots	Peas	
Broccoli	Oatmeal	
Swiss chard	Nuts	
Kale		
Peaches		
Spinach		
Yellow squash		
Asparagus		
Cantaloupe		
Dandelion greens		
Mustard greens		
Red peppers		
Spirulina		
Turnip greens		
Watercress		

VITAMIN B2 (THIAMIN)	VITAMIN B6 (PYRIDOXINE)	VITAMIN B12 (CYANOCOBALAMIN)
Beans	Brewer's yeast	Tofu
Asparagus	Carrots	
Avocados	Peas	
Brussel sprouts	Spinach	
Currants	Sunflower seeds	
Nuts	Walnuts	
	Wheat germ	

INOSITOL	FOLIC ACID	VITAMIN B3 (RIBOFLAVIN)
Fruits	Yeast	Almonds
Vegetables	Barley	Broccoli
Whole grains	Beans	Carrots
	Bran	Corn flour
	Brewer's yeast	Potatoes
	Brown rice	Tomatoes
	Dates	Whole wheat
	Green leafy veg.	Sunflower seeds
	Lentils	Peanuts
	Oranges	
	Split peas	
	Wheat germ	

CHOLINE	PABA	VITAMIN C
Legumes	Molasses	Green vegetables
Whole grain cereals	Whole grains	Berries
		Citrus fruits

VITAMIN K	COENZYME Q10	BORON
Alfalfa	Spinach	Green leafy veg.
Broccoli	Peanuts	Fruits
Green leafy veg.		Nuts
Soybeans		Grains
Vitamin E		
Cold-pressed veg. oils		

VITAMIN K (CON'T)	LYCOPENE FOODS
Whole Grains	Tomatoes
Nuts And Seeds	Watermelons
Legumes	Guavas
Dry Beans	Papayas
Mangos	Apricots
Wheat Germ	Pink Grapefruits

CALCIUM	CHROMIUM (GTF)	COPPER
Green leafy veg.	Brewer's yeast	Almonds
Almonds	Brown rice	Avocados
Asparagus	Whole grains	Barley
Blackstrap molasses	Dried beans	Beans
Brewer's yeast	Mushrooms	Beet roots
Broccoli	Potatoes	Blackstrap molasses
Cabbage		Broccoli
Carob		Dandelion greens
Collards		Garlic
Figs		Lentils
Dulse		Mushrooms
Kelp		Nuts
Sesame seeds		Oats
Tofu		Oranges
		Radishes
		Raisins
		Soybeans
		Green leafy veg.

GERMANIUM (GE-132)	IODINE	MANGANESE
Aloe vera	Kelp	Avocados
Comfrey		Nuts and seeds
Garlic		Seaweed
Shitake mushrooms		Whole grains
Onions		

IRON	POTASSIUM	PHYTOCHEMICAL FOODS
Green leafy veg.	Apricots	Soybeans
Whole grains	Avocados	Soy products
Almonds	Bananas	Hot chili peppers
Millet	Blackstrap molasses	Tomatoes
Parsley	Brewer's yeast	Broccoli
Peaches	Brown rice	Citrus fruits
Pears	Dates	Berries
Dried prunes	Figs	Apricots
Pumpkins	Broccoli	Garlic
Raisins	Garlic	Onions
Rice and wheat bran	Nuts	Grapes
Sesame seeds	Potatoes	Oats
Soybeans	Raisins	Watermelons
Avocados	Winter squash	Pomegranates
Beets	Wheat bran	Cherries
Brewer's yeast	Yams	Apples
Dates	Chard	Herbs
Dulse	Spinach	Spices
Kelp	Romaine	Garlic
Kidney beans	Mustard greens	Cruciferous veg.
Lima beans	Fennel bulb	Flax seeds
Lentils	Cauliflower	Beans
		Grains and seeds

ANTIOXIDANT FOODS	LUTEIN FOODS	BIOFLAVANOIDS
Yams	Collard greens	Citrus fruits
Endive	Spinach	Fruits
Butternut squash	Kale	Peppers
Apricots		Buckwheat
Winter squash		Black currants
Mangos		
Pumpkins		
Papayas		
Carrots		
Cantaloupe		
Spinach		
Tomatoes		
Broccoli		

SURPRISING NUTRIENTS FOUND IN FRUITS AND VEGETABLES

CALCIUM	PROTEIN	IRON
Blackberries	Tamari (soy sauce)	Thyme
Papaya	Mustard greens	Cumin
Carrot	Romaine lettuce	Basil
Celery	Crimini mushrooms	Cinnamon
Endive	Asparagus	Oregano
Lemon	Broccoli	Turmeric
Orange	Chard	Black pepper
Turnip	Cauliflower	Romaine lettuce
Watercress	Cabbage	Peppermint leaves
Parsley	Shiitake mushrooms	String beans
Nuts and seeds	Turnip greens	Dried beans
Chickpeas	Mustard seeds	Whole wheat
Yellow wax beans	Summer squash	Dried peas
	Pumpkin seeds	Celery
	Garlic	Spinach
	Tomato	Figs
		Turnips
		Tomatoes
		Cabbage
		Mustard greens
		Shiitake mushrooms
		Turnip greens
		String beans
		Kale
		Brussel sprouts
		Asparagus

ZINC

Crimini mushrooms
Asparagus
Parsley
Summer squash
Collard greens
Miso (soybeans)
Seeds
Lentils
Tofu
Green beans

Sarena S. Johnson

MEAL PLAN GUIDE
THE BASIC FOUR

Fruits
Vegetables
Whole Grains and Legumes
Proteins and Fats
(Nuts, Seeds, Oils)

VEGETARIANS (NO MEAT)
1. Vegetables
2. Fruits
3. Whole grains/legumes
4. Nuts and seeds
Food Group Priorities—(1=eat most often, 4=least)

MEAT EATERS
1. Vegetables
2. Fruits
3. Whole grains/legumes
4. Nuts and seeds
5. Poultry/wild game (or tested freshwater fish), free-range, organic
6. Dairy, organic, raw is best
Food Group Priorities—(1=eat most often, 6=least)

Avoid eating all fish, unless you know the fish has been tested and shown not to contain harmful levels of mercury and other toxins. (Check label or contact company.)

SUMMARY

1. If trying to lose weight limit whole grains/legumes. Vegetables and fruits (those higher in water content, (like grapes, oranges, etc.), should be the largest part of your meals. Limit nuts and seeds. Eat grains early in the day (breakfast, lunch, mid-afternoon.)

2. Use fruit as dessert.

3. Don't eat three hours before bed. If you need to eat, choose a vegetable or fruit.

4. Get sleep! Sleep deficiency will cause you to eat more, work less efficiently (burn fewer calories), and have a bad attitude!

5. Drink lots of water. Dehydration will cause you to want food when you are not hungry.

6. If eating packaged foods, look for foods with a small number of ingredients, whole-food sources (whole oats), and natural preservatives (vitamin E).

7. Take supplements—we can not get all nutritional requirements from the food we eat today. I recommend a comprehensive multivitamin/antioxidant formula along with a pure fish-oil supplement (tested for mercury and toxins) to get your needed essential fatty acids.

8. If you eat meat, consider it a luxury item to eat on special occasions.

The above information is a guide and may need to be changed according to your body's individual needs.

NOTES

BODY BEVERAGE

THE MOST IMPORTANT BEVERAGE FOR YOUR HEALTH
IS WATER. MORE IMPORTANTLY, FILTERED WATER. DUE TO THE
POLLUTANTS IN OUR WATER SUPPLY, I RECOMMEND DRINKING FILTERED WATER.
IT IS REALLY HARD TO DETERMINE THE AMOUNT OF WATER TO DRINK FOR
EVERY PERSON. I BELIEVE MOST PEOPLE DO NOT DRINK ENOUGH WATER OR
WATER-CONTAINING DRINKS/FOODS. I RECOMMEND YOU DRINK OFTEN.
YOUR URINE SHOULD BE VERY LIGHT YELLOW TO CLEAR IF YOU ARE
HYDRATED. DEHYDRATION WILL CAUSE YOU TO FEEL TIRED,
EAT MORE, AND NOT OPERATE EFFICIENTLY.

8

CRACKING THE CODE TO HEALTHY FOOD SHOPPING

BY NOW YOU know I suggest a whole-foods diet. In this chapter, you will find suggestions for healthier processed foods to substitute for the "American Standard Diet." My recommendation is to choose whole-grain and whole-food products such as fruits, vegetables, beans, and rice for your daily consumption and eat the "healthier processed" foods on special occasions such as school snacks, picnics, parties, etc.

Cost is a subject that comes up often when families are switching from the Standard American Diet to healthier food choices. My answer to the cost question is simply—it ends up costing you less when you stop buying all the extra "junk" (chips, cookies, candy, hot dogs, whip cream, ice cream, soda, etc.)! Even if you stick to store brand "oatmeal"—and add bananas—it is a better choice than a processed packet of "Apple and Oats" or other "candy cereal." It is also less expensive when you consider the price your body is paying in energy deficiency, sickness, and all the medications you will someday need from eating poorly.

Whether you choose to buy organic or non-organic (I have included some of both) foods, look for whole foods, such as brown rice, oatmeal, etc. Try to find foods without added sugar or salt (it is hard—but possible). If an ingredients label has a paragraph larger than this and you can't pronounce the ingredient names—don't buy it!

Beware! Manufacturers will change their ingredients without notice so be sure to read your favorite food labels periodically. If a manufacturer makes a "health food" don't assume all their products are good products or contain the same type of ingredients.

I have not listed foods labeled with the common "evaporated cane juice/cane juice/naturally milled sugar" as "health food" aisles are loaded with them. Avoid or limit these foods.

I have divided food categories into: breakfast; lunch and dinner; snacks; condiments; no added sugar or salt; no sugar or salt.

SHOPPING TIPS

- Soy meat can be highly processed and may contain salt, sugar (various types), preservatives, dairy, and additives—read the ingredients.

- Organic frozen fruit is a good alternative in the winter.

- If you buy dairy, meat, or eggs look for organic, free-range (or better yet buy organic "raw" from a local farm).

- Buy unprocessed, raw foods when available—including vinegar and honey.

- Look for non-GMO foods.

- If foods don't contain sugar, they often contain salt. Try to use "sea salt" as much as possible. Look for foods (even if you are to get foods with organic cane sugar) containing 7 grams or less of sugar per serving unless they contain natural sugars from fruit.

- Foods are frequently added to the "health food" market. The information in this book provides you necessary tools to discriminate between good, healthy foods and those that aren't.

BREAKFAST

Non-Dairy Milk—rice, soy, and almond (Westbrae Westsoy Organics Low-Fat Plain; Eden Foods—EdenBlend Rice & Soy; Original; Edensoy Extra)

Bread (Food for Life—Ezekiel Breads, except Bran for Life; French Meadow Bakery)

Cold Cereals (Arrowhead Mills Spelt Flakes; Food for Life—Ezekiel 4:9 Almond, Ezekiel 4:9 Original, Ezekiel 4:9 Golden Flax, Ezekiel 4:9 Cinnamon Raisin; Barbara's Bakery—Breakfast O's, Brown Rice Crisps, Corn Flakes, Puffins Cinnamon; Nature's Path—Organic Corn Flakes,

Millet Rice; Cascadian Farms Purely O's; Erewhon—Crispy Brown Rice, Corn Flakes, Crispy Brown Rice with Mixed Berries, Whole Wheat Flakes, Raisin Bran, Fruit and Wheat, Kamut Flakes, Apple Stroodles, Aztec; Breadshop's Granola; Kashi—Seven in the Morning, Pufffed Kashi Seven Whole Grains and Sesame)

Pancake Mix (Arrowhead Mills)

LUNCH AND DINNER

Soups (Imagine, Pacific)

Tortillas, Pitas, Mufffins, etc. (Garden of Eatin', Food For Life, French Meadow Bakery)

Soy Burgers/Meat Substitutes (Amy's—California Burger; Turtle Island Tofurkey—lots of products; Hearty & Natural—Wild Mushroom Burger, Mexican Red Bean Burger)

Cheese (Some have lots of salt and cane sugar/juice—read labels.)

> **Non-Dairy** (Soya Kaas and Soymage by Galaxy Foods, Lisanatti)

> **Soy Free**—Rice, Almond, and Oat (Galaxy Foods)

SNACKS

Seeds—Sesame, Sunflower, etc. (Arrowhead Mills)

Cookies (Tree of Life, Mrs. Denson's, Nana's)

Crackers—Animal (Barbara's Snackimals—Vanilla Only, Healthy Times); "Crispbread" type (Wasa); Oyster (Hain)

Pretzels (Paul Newman)

Chips/Sticks (Naturally Preferred, Guiltless Gourmet, Michael Seasons, Eden, Good Health, Terra, Kettle, Genisoy Soy Crisps—Deep Sea Salted, Roberts American Gourmet—Super veggie Tings, Blue Chips, Awesome Party Chips, Veggie Booty, Fruity Booty—some are very high in fat so check the labels!)

100% Fruit Snacks (Stretch Island)

Dried Fruit—raisins, dates, figs, prunes, etc. (Earthbound Farms, Sunview, Naturally Preferred, Good For Life-Premiere Valley Foods, Inc., Made in Nature)

Fig Bars (Barbara's)

Bars (Nature's Choice—Cereal Bars, Granola Peanut Butter Bars; Nana's)

CONDIMENTS AND MISC.

Mustard (Eden)

Soy Mayonnaise—and other "mayo" type condiments (Spectrum Naturals, Earth Island Veganaise)

Sea Salt (Redmond Real Salt, DeSouza's Solar Sea Salt, Frontier Unrefined Sea Salt)

100% Fruit Spreads (Tree of Life, St. Balfour, Margie's, Wild Oats, Bionature)

Bean Dips (Guiltless Gourmet, Dessert Pepper)

Salsa (Muir Glen, Green Mountain Gringo, Drew's, Dessert Pepper Trading Co., Seeds of Change, Enrico's, Wild Oats)

Pasta Sauce (Amy's—Family Marinara ONLY, Eden Organic, Wild Oats)

Pure Maple Syrup (Up Country Organics, Spring Tree Organic, Shady Maple Farms, Wild Oats)

Soy Margarine (Soy Garden, Earth Balance)

Dressings (Nasoya, Annie's, Up Country Organics, Wild Oats)

Baking Powder (non-aluminum—Rumford, Featherweight)

Baking Soda (Bob's Red Mill)

Oils—-Olive, flax, almond, etc. (International Collection, Boyajian, Spectrum Naturals, Rapunzel, Iliada, Bionature, Colavita, DeCarla, Arrowhead Mills, Nature's Way, Barlean's, Eden)

Organic Spices (The Spice Hunter)

Pure Vanilla Extract—Alcohol-free (Frontier)

Caffeine Free Tea—Make sure they are caffeine-free and contain no sugar. (Celestial Seasonings, Traditional

Medicine, Brassica, Choice Organ Tea)

Vinegar—Apple cider, rice, balsamic (Bragg's, Newman's Own, Eden, Spectrum Naturals, Hain)

Honey—Raw, local, unprocessed (local farm or health food store.)

Rapadura (Rapunzel)

FOODS WITH NO ADDED SALT OR SUGAR

Below are foods that do not contain added salt or sugar but may contain naturally occurring salt or sugar. Look for the words "No Salt/Sugar Added" or "Unsalted." I have listed only foods that are packaged (not whole-foods such as fruits and vegetables).

Sauce—Apple, cherry, etc. (Mott's Unsweetened, Leroux Creek Cinnamon Applesauce, Santa Cruz Apple Cherry Sauce, Eden Organic, Garden of Eatin', Solana Gold Organic)

Bread (Nature's Path Manna Bread)

Nut Butters (Krema; Marantha—Organic Roasted Tahini, Almond; Arrowhead Mills—Peanut, Tahini; Kettle—Sesame, Peanut, Cashew; East Wind; Rejuvenative Foods; Spanky's)

Carob Powder (Chatfields)

Pasta (Hodgson Mill, Bella Terra, Eddies, Deboles, Mrs. Leeper's, Naturally Preferred, Annie's, Bionature, Tinkya'da)

Pasta Sauce (Wild Oats Pepper)

Lentils & Beans (Eden Organic)

Whole Brown Rice (Lundberg, Kroger, Meijer, etc.)

Crackers (Bran a Crisp)

Soy Sauce (Bragg's Liquid Amino Acid)

Chips (Michael Season's Unsalted, Guiltless Gourmet No Salt and Unsalted, Garden of Eatin' No Salt Added)

Soybeans (Seapoint Farm Shelled Soybeans, Edamame Soybeans in a pod)

Tofu (Soy Deli, Nasoya Lite Tofu, White Wave, Spring Creek)

Fruit (Cascadian Farms)

Soy Milk (Silk Unsweetened Soy Milk by White Wave)

FOODS WITH NO SALT OR SUGAR

These foods do not contain any added salt or sugar or naturally occurring salt or sugar.

Soy Milk (WestSoy Unsweetened Soy Milk)

Tofu (Nasoya [Not Lite] and Soy Deli)

Soybeans (Seapoint Farms No Salt Added)

Hot Cereals (Arrowhead Mills, Erewhon, Mother's, Barbara's Bakery, Kashi Company, Lundberg, Quaker Oats, U.S. Mills, Bob's Red Mill, Kroger (Oats, Regular),

Country Choice, Mother's, McCannes Irish Oatmeal, Hodgson Mills)

Brown Rice Cakes (Mother's—Unsalted Plain, Unsalted Sesame, Lundberg Brown Rice Cakes)

Cold Cereal (Barbara's Bakery Original Shredded Wheat)

Flours & Grains (Arrowhead Mills, King Arthur, Hodgson Mills, Bob's Red Mill)

Brown Rice (Lundberg, Texmati, lots of brands)

Green Foods—Spinach, barley, etc. (Organic by Nature, Earthbound Farms, etc.)

NOTES

"THOU SHOULDST EAT TO LIVE NOT LIVE TO EAT."
—SOCRATES (469 BC - 399 BC)

QUICK TIPS

- Plastic leaches into foods, especially oils, so try to get glass bottles.
- Cook foods in the microwave in glass.
- The more cloudy the honey, the better.
- Crystallized honey is best!

APPENDICES

1

RECIPE TIPS AND SUBSTITUTIONS

T HIS CHAPTER IS designed to give you healthy nutrition
tips and substitutions for cooking and baking.

QUICK MEASUREMENT EQUIVALENTS

5gms.=1tsp.
3tsp.=1T.=15gms.=.5oz.
30gms.=1oz.
16T.=1C.=8oz.
1/8C.=1oz.=2T.
8oz.=1C.
2C.=1 pint
32oz.=4C.=1qt.=2 pints
64oz.=8C.=2qt.=4 pints= 1/2 gallon

RECIPE SUBSTITUTES

USE:	INSTEAD OF:	NOTES:
Pure Maple Syrup	White sugar	Use 2/3-1/4 C for 1 C. white sugar. Reduce liquid in recipe by 3 Tbsp. and add 1/4 tsp. of baking soda per cup of maple syrup.
Rapadura	White sugar	Replace equal amounts for sugar. Add 1/4 tsp. baking soda per cup.
Honey	White sugar	Use ½ less than sugar. Reduce liquids in recipe by 1/4 C. If there is no liquid to reduce, add 3-4 Tbsp. of flour for each 1/2 honey used. Add 1/8 tsp. honey per ½ honey used. Lower baking temp. 25 degrees and adjust time.
Barley Malt (use in spiced foods such as cakes, cookies, and gingerbread.)	White sugar	Substitute 1 1/3 C. for every 1 C. white sugar called for in recipe. Reduce liquid by 1/4 C. and add 1/4 tsp. baking soda per cup rice syrup used.
Brown Rice Syrup (use in cookies, crisps, granola, pies, and puddings. Do not use in cakes or any type of bread—produces a gooey center).	White sugar	
Silken Tofu Soy Yogurt	Butter	Equal amounts

USE:	INSTEAD OF:	NOTES:
Pureed prunes (Baby food—Earth's Best)	Butter	1/2 the amount of fat in recipes that would allow the taste (great with anything requiring chocolate, carrot cake or gingerbread)
3/4 C. chopped, pitted prunes + 3 Tbsp. boiling water	Baby food prunes	
Tofu + Soy Yogurt or Tofu Sour Cream	Sour cream	
3 Tbsp. Carob Powder + 1 oz. Olive Oil or Soy Margarine. Reduce sugar by 1/4.	Unsweetened baking chocolate	
Crumbled Tofu	Ricotta cheese	
1 C. Soy Milk + 2 Tbsp. Lemon Juice or White Vinegar	Buttermilk	
Corn starch	Gelatin	
Olive oil	Lard	
Portabella Mushrooms, Tofu, Beans, or Tempeh	Meat	
Soy Milk + 1 Tbsp. Olive Oil	Whole milk	
Carob Chips or Powder	Chocolate	
1/2 C. Soy Milk + 1/2 C. Tofu	Heavy cream	
Applesauce	Oil	Also a replacement for egg, add 1/2 tsp. baking soda
1/2 Mashed Banana	1 Egg	

USE:	INSTEAD OF:	NOTES:
1/4 C. pureed Silken Tofu Increase Baking Powder 1/4-1/2 tsp.,	1 Egg	
1/2 tsp. Baking Powder + 2 Tbsp. Liquid	1 Egg	
1/4 tsp. Baking Soda + Acidic Liquid (lemon, vinegar, etc)	1 tsp. baking powder	

QUICK TIPS

- Baking powder is 1/4 baking soda with dry acid and powder fillers added (corn starch).
- Double-acting baking powder contains baking soda plus two dry acids. You get leavening when the liquid is added and again when the mixture is heated (with single-acting it is either/or).
- Baking soda can be substituted for baking powder (1/4 teaspoon to 1 teaspoon) as long as there is an acidic liquid in the mix.
- If you are substituting a liquid sweetener for a dry sweetener (such as honey for sugar), decrease liquids by 1/4 cup per cup of sweetener or add 1/4 cup of flour. Add 1/2 tsp baking soda per 1 cup of liquid to counteract the acidity. Decrease baking powder by 2 teaspoons or eliminate it.[1]
- If buying baking powder make sure it is aluminum free.
- No applesauce? Peel an apple; add water; puree with hand mixer.
- When you see "tofu" in baking recipes you generally want to use soft or silken tofu (good for drinks too). Silken works better in most recipes (and drinks)—try both and see what you like.

NOTES

"WHAT IT LIES IN OUR POWER TO DO, IT LIES IN OUR POWER NOT TO DO."
—ARISTOTLE

2

Logs and Forms

Action Diary
Goal-Setting Form
Contract to Change
Food Log
Grocery Store Log

THESE LOGS ARE designed to help you determine why you are eating your current "diet," and how your body reacts to those foods, both physically (through energy, skin rash, headaches, digestion, etc.) and mentally (through depression, moods, self-esteem, mental focus, etc).

If necessary, keep your own journal. This is not something that you have to do consistently, but it's a great tool to help you become aware of how your body reacts to food.

The more nutrient dense "good foods" you feed your body, the fewer cravings you will have for "bad foods." You will also be more in tune with how foods (and other products) affect your body.

ACTION DIARY

1   What actions control my life?

_____

_____

_____

_____

2   What are my priorities?

_____

_____

_____

_____

_____

3   What are my goals? (see Goal-Setting Form)

_____

_____

_____

_____

_____

4 What do people see in you or know about you?

_____

_____

_____

_____

_____

5 What do you want them to see?

_____

_____

_____

_____

_____

6 What actions do you need to change to become that person?

_____

_____

_____

_____

_____

7 Why do you want to change?*

_____

_____

_____

_____

*A key element in permanent change is accepting responsibility for your actions and deciding to change. If your weight and/or health "problems" are always due to "genetics," "children," "notime," "my family," etc., then you will never change. Even if some "barriers" are hindering your efforts, they do not control you or your outcome. You and only you are in control of your eating, exercise, and health. Until you take responsibility, your weight and health may never change. In addition, if you are losing weight or improving your nutrition habits to please other people—not because you want to—your attempts may be unsuccessful.

MORE ACTION STRATEGIES

Changing your lifestyle is dependent on changing your thinking, which in turn changes your actions. Your mind is a powerful force in any life matter.

Combat your (or someone else's) negative self-talk with positive self-talk. Know that your health matters because you matter. This is a big barrier between women and health. They think (wrongly!) that health is not worth it because they are not worth it. Please don't think that. Anytime you ever think or hear those words, STOP! Change your words (or leave the room if it is someone else!). YOU ARE WORTH IT!

When you find yourself in the middle of a bad habit, STOP! Interrupt the habit by replacing it with something else. Our actions are habitual. They will need to be replaced with healthy habits and repeated over time to change.

Finally, what works for someone else may not work for you. As stated earlier, everybody is created a little differently. She may need more nutrients and calories than you. His body may handle foods differently than yours. Everyone is unique in his or her needs. Listen to your body.

NOTES

As Einstein always said, "The imagination is a far greater asset than the mind." Change starts from your deep desire to know you can do it—and know you are worth it! Remember the "It Principle."

GOAL-SETTING DIRECTIONS

1. *Lifestyle goals* are what you ultimately want to accomplish. They are detailed and have a "goal date." For instance, I want to reduce my body fat from 35 percent to 20 percent in one year (whatever the date is a year from now).

2. *Intermediate goals* are short-term goals you are going to accomplish to meet your long-term goal (between now and your long-term goal date).

3. *Process goals* are short-term "action" steps to help you achieve your intermediate and long-term goals. This is the most important step! If you want to succeed, keep your focus on your path (even narrow it to everyday actions)! Examples are: Eliminate red meat. Eliminate dairy. Eat five servings of vegetables today.

4. Examples of potential barriers to achieving long-term goals and strategies to overcome them are:

Barrier: Easily blow off exercise.
Strategy: Schedule exercise with a partner who will make you accountable.
Barrier: Too much junk food around the house.
Strategy: Throw it away. If it's not there, you can't eat it!

Barriers can be people, food, exercise, time, will power—anything that prohibits you from reaching your goal.

GOAL-SETTING FORM

Long-Term Goal (s) (include goal dates)

1_____

2_____

3_____

A Intermediate Goals (include goal dates)

1_____

2_____

3_____

B Process Goals

1 1 month

_____

_____

_____

_____

2 3 months

_____

_____

_____

_____

3 6 months

_____

_____

_____

_____

Potential barriers to achieving long-term goals:

1_____

Strategy to overcome barrier:

_____

_____

_____

_____

2_____

Strategy to overcome barrier:

_____

_____

_____

_____

3_____

Strategy to overcome barrier:

_____

_____

_____

_____

BEFORE PICTURE

Place your "before" picture here or describe in picture words.

GOAL PICTURE

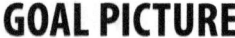

PLACE YOUR "GOAL" PICTURE HERE OR DESCRIBE IN PICTURE WORDS (USE AS MUCH DETAIL AS POSSIBLE).

Think about your goals and the consequences if you do not take action. Do you want to continue down the same path? Do you want to live your life the way you are today?

To further your commitment I would like you to sign the contract on the following page. Have your spouse or friend sign it too. Include a reward you will give yourself if you reach your goal (trip, shopping for new clothes, new gym equipment, etc.).

Keep in mind that eating too much, missing your exercise appointment, "falling off the wagon" for a week—these are not failures. If this happens, don't be discouraged, it happens to everyone. It's not what happens in a day or week—but over time. Keep on keeping on. If you eat too much one day, cut back the next. If you "fall off the wagon" one week, begin your routine the next. This is a life change not a diet. Think of your goals. Think of the freedom.

CONTRACT TO CHANGE

I, _____, hereby agree to achieve the above goal(s) by the dates specified.

I realize that if I do, it will change my life dramatically—both during the process, and for the rest of my life.

If the goal(s) are obtained as stated above, I will receive the following as a reward:

_____

_____

_____

_____

Life-Changer Signature

_____

Witness Signature

"WE MUST BECOME THE CHANGE WE WANT TO SEE."
—MAHATMA GANDHI (1869 - 1948)

FOOD LOG AND DIARY

Time of Day	Food/ Beverage (banana, Coke)	How Much (oz./ quantity)	Physical Feeling (sluggish, tired, headache, no energy, bloating)	Mental Feeling (mood swings, can't concentrate, depressed)

GROCERY LOG

Store Name _____

Food Name	Made by	Aisle	Notes

NOTES

"WHEN IT IS A QUESTION OF GOD'S ALMIGHTY SPIRIT, NEVER SAY,
"'I CAN'T.'"
—OSWALD CHAMBERS

3

THE SECRET TO A HEALTHY
MIND, BODY, AND SPIRIT

WOULDN'T IT BE great if you could get advice from someone who knows everything about the subject you are inquiring about? You can! Our Creator has left us a "manual" for every aspect of our lives (health, love, happiness, work, family, etc.). This "manual" is called the Bible. In it God reveals Himself and His wisdom. The Bible states: "All Scripture is inspired by God and is useful to teach us what is true and to make us realize what is wrong in our lives. It straightens us out and teaches us to do what is right.

It is God's way of preparing us in every way, fully equipped for every good thing God wants us to do." (2 Timothy 3:16-17, NLT)

One of the greatest messages God reveals to us in the Bible is that we can have abundant life through a personal relationship with Him. This relationship is called salvation. We need salvation because of our sinful nature. Because of our sinful nature we are separated from God and have no hope. The Bible states, "For all have sinned and fall short of the Glory of God." (Romans 3:23, NKJV)

The wonderful news is that because God loves us so much He created a way for us to be restored to a personal relationship with Him. "God so loved the world that He gave his only begotten Son, that whoever believes in Him should not perish but have everlasting life." (John 3:16, KJV). God Himself came to earth in the Person of Jesus Christ. He was crucified, died, was buried, and arose from the dead. He suffered so we can have an abundant life. A life filled with health, happiness, and hope.

"He personally carried away our sins in his own body on the cross so we can be dead to sin and live for what is right. You have been healed by his wounds." (1 Peter 2:24, NLT) "For what I received I passed on to you, as of first importance: that Christ died for our sins according to the Scriptures, that he was buried, that he was raised on the third day according to the Scriptures..." (1 Corinthians 14:36, NIV).

Do you feel hopeless? Do you feel like you live without a purpose? God created you for a purpose. "For I know the plans I have for you," declares the Lord. "Plans to prosper you and not to harm you, plans to give you hope and a future." (Jeremiah 29:11, NIV)

He is waiting for a relationship with you. It is something you must choose. You must do the following:

1. Admit you need Him and are a sinner.

2. Repent and turn from your sin. You are turning away from your sins (repenting) and your way of doing things and turning to Him and His way of doing things.

3. Believe that Jesus Christ died for you on the Cross and arose from the grave.

4. Receive Jesus Christ into your heart and life. Trust Jesus and only Him to save you.

"Behold, I stand at the door, and knock: if any man hear my voice, and open the door, I will come to him..." (Revelation 3:20, KJV)

"If you confess with your mouth the Lord Jesus and believe in your heart that God has raised Him from the dead you will be saved." (Romans 10:9, NKJV)

All you have to do is pray. Prayer is just talking to God. Pray from your heart. If you need help here is an example. "Jesus, I know that I am a sinner and need your forgiveness. I have been living for me and I want to live for you. I want to turn from my sins. I believe that you died on the cross for my sins, and that you arose from the grave. I now ask you to forgive me of my sins and come into my heart as my Lord and Savior. Amen."

It is my desire that you live a life of incredible love, peace, health, and happiness. That you trust your soul to the One who loves you so much that He created you and provides instructions for your health and happiness in the Bible.

NOTES

"THE STRENGTH OF A MAN CONSISTS IN FINDING OUT THE WAY
GOD IS GOING, AND GOING THAT WAY."
—HENRY WARD BEECHER

4

NUTRITION STUDIES AND FACTS

MEAT, DAIRY, EGGS
VEGETABLES AND FRUIT
SEEDS, NUTS, AND BEANS
SUGAR
MEAT, DAIRY, AND EGGS

I N THE BOOK, *God's Way to Ultimate Health, A Common Sense Guide for Eliminating Sickness Through Nutrition,*[1] Dr. George H. Malkmus states, "The facts are that meat, dairy, and eggs can be linked directly or indirectly to 90 percent of all physical problems and deaths in America today!!!"

I don't believe God gave us food that would make us so sick. What I believe is that we have taken God's natural foods and loaded them with fat, hormones, chemicals, toxins, and diseases and then consumed these foods in larger quantities than intended. Additionally, manufacturers take chemical, fat-laden milk products and pasteurize and homogenize them—destroying the beneficial nutrients—causing them to have to add or "enrich" them.

You never read about high protein diets (or any diets!) in the Bible. You read about natural grains, fruits, vegetables, fish, and other meats (whole foods). You will see two radically different scenarios when you compare Biblical times verses today:

1. They ate meat occasionally—not every meal.

2. Their animals were lean and free-range.

Today you will find animals (all, not just cows) in cramped cages loaded with hormones for greater quantities of milk, meat, and egg production and in unsanitary conditions. Over the years, numerous studies have confirmed the problems associated with dairy, milk, and egg products:

1. CANCER

Red meat and fat consumption appears to be associated with colon cancer, the second-leading cause of cancer death in the United States, a disease that strikes women and men at about the same rate.[2]

A study of the Seventh-Day Adventists, who eat little red meat and animal fat, found that they had about half the rate of colon cancer as the general population. They also refrain, however, from drinking alcohol and smoking, which may also contribute to their better health.[3]

A separate, ongoing study by the Harvard School of Public Health involving 89,000 nurses found that those who ate the most animal fat were almost twice as likely to develop colon cancer as those who ate the least. The nurses who ate skinless chicken or fish instead of beef, pork or lamb, cut their risk by 50%.[3]

At least two studies also have linked high-fiber, low-fat diets to a significant reduction in the number of precancerous colon and rectal polyps. It is speculated that fiber moves through the colon faster and, as a result, limits the exposure of the colon wall to carcinogenic substances.[3]

The American Cancer Society also says that high-fat diets, especially those high in red meat, have been linked to increased prostate cancer.[3]

In one study of 48,000 male health professionals ages 40 to 75, it was found that those who ate the highest amount of fat had 79 percent more cases of advanced prostate cancer, according to the *New Wellness Encyclopedia* from the University of California at Berkeley. Those who ate the most red meat had a 164 percent higher incidence of advanced prostate cancer than those who ate the least.

Consequently, the American Cancer Society, citing the colon and prostate cancer link, came out with dietary guidelines recommending that people limit their intake of red meat and consume more fruits, vegetables, and whole grains.

DID YOU KNOW?

A number of people think chicken is healthier than red meat. Chicken has the same amount of cholesterol as beef and is loaded with growth hormones.[4]

2. OSTEOPOROSIS

Not only does cow's milk have enough fat to turn a 45-pound calf into a 400-pound cow but it can cause osteoporosis. Yes, you read it right. You have been told over and over again that you need the calcium in cow's milk for healthy bones. This, too, is false.

Even studies paid for by the National Dairy Council have shown that the excessive protein in milk lowers blood calcium levels, causing the body to draw on calcium from the bones. The result is that milk drinkers have much higher incidences of osteoporosis than vegans who drink no milk and eat no meat!

In fact, osteoporosis is virtually unheard of among vegans. African Bantu women average only 350 milligrams calcium per day. They also average the birth of nine children, each of whom they breast feed for two years. Yet they never suffer from calcium deficiency. Osteoporosis is almost nonexistent, even in women over 65 years of age.

In contrast Inuit Eskimos consume 3500 milligrams of calcium each day, and are crippled by the disease.[5] Below are further studies.

i. In 1994, the *American Journal of Epidemiology* (volume 139)[6] reported: "Consumption of dairy products, particularly at age 20 years, was associated with an increased risk of hip fractures...metabolism of dietary protein causes increased urinary excretion of calcium."

ii. "In 1988, N.A. Breslau and colleagues identified the relationship between protein-rich diets and calcium metabolism, noting that protein caused calcium loss. His work was published in the *Journal of Clinical Endocrinology* (1988;66:140-6)."[6]

iii. A 1994 study published in the *American Journal of Clinical Nutrition* (Remer T, Am J Clin. Nutr. 1994;59:1356-61) found that animal proteins cause calcium to be leached from the bones and excreted in the urine.[6]

iv. "A study published in the January, 2001 edition of the *American Journal of Clinical Nutrition* examined the diets of 1,035 women, particularly focusing on the protein intake from animal and vegetable products. Deborah Sellmeyer, M.D., found: ANIMAL PROTEIN INCREASES BONE LOSS. In her study, women with a high animal-to-vegetable protein ratio experienced an increased rate of femoral neck bone loss. A high animal-to-vegetable protein ratio was also associated with an increased risk of hip fracture... How ironic it is that the dairy industry continues to promote the cause of bone disease as the cure."[7]

vi. "Milk does not protect against bone breaks." The Harvard Nurses' Health Study, including 77,761 women, aged 34 to 59 and followed for 12 years, showed that those who got more calcium from milk actually had slightly, but significantly, more fractures, compared to those who drank little or no milk.[8]

vii. A 1994 study of elderly men and women in Sydney, Australia, showed much the same thing—higher dairy product consumption was associated with increased fracture risk. Those with the highest dairy product consumption had approximately double the risk of hip fracture, compared to those with the lowest consumption.[8]

This does not mean that calcium is not important. Dairy products do not protect against bone fractures, according to the best evidence we have. Good nondairy sources of calcium include green leafy vegetables, beans, almonds, carob, cabbage, figs, kale, kelp, sesame seeds, tofu, oats, and prunes. Just as important, reducing sodium (salt) intake, avoiding animal protein, and quitting smoking helps your body keep calcium where it belongs instead of losing it through the kidneys into the urine.

DO YOU KNOW THE HEALTH OF YOUR MEAT?...

"If you don't finish your steak at a restaurant, did you know the leftovers might be dinner for a cow? Or that calves, instead of drinking their mothers' milk, are fed formula made from cows' blood? These practices, all perfectly legal…Americans have a bucolic image of cows happily chomping grass in fields. Many don't know that modern animal husbandry practices have provided cheap, plentiful meat through such standard practices as feeding cattle not only pieces of their herd mates (before the practice was banned in 1997) but also chicken litter, leftover restaurant food and out-of-date pet food."[2]

...OR YOUR MILK?

Resistance to tuberculosis increased in children fed raw milk instead of pasteurized, to the point that in five years only one case of pulmonary TB had developed, whereas in the previous five years, when children had been given pasteurized milk, fourteen cases of pulmonary TB had developed.

FRUITS AND VEGETABLES

Epidemiological studies have repeatedly shown that populations whose diets include plenty of fruits and vegetables have lower rates of cancer, heart disease, and other "ailments of aging." That's why fruits and vegetables are high on the list of recommended foods in the Dietary Guidelines for Americans.[10]

The Journal of the American Dietetic Association states, "Epidemiologic evidence of a protective role for fruits and vegetables in cancer prevention is substantial."[11]

SEEDS, NUTS, AND BEANS

In a recent study at the Division of Urologic Surgery at Duke University, 25 prostate cancer patients were placed on a short term (34 days average) low-fat diet supplemented with flaxseed and its lignan component. The researchers reported differences in the biology of the tumors. "Tumor cells (of men on the diet and supplementation) did not divide as quickly and there was a greater rate of apoptosis (tumor cell reduction) in this group," noted Dr. Demark-Wahnefried, lead researcher.[12]

Dietary fat and fiber can affect hormone levels and may influence cancer progression. Flaxseed is high in fiber and is the richest source of plant-based, omega-3 fatty acids. Studies suggest that dietary fiber reduces cancer risk, and omega-3 fatty acids also have shown a protective benefit against cancer. Flaxseed is also a rich source of lignan, a specific family of fiber-related compounds that appear to play an important role in influencing both estrogen and androgen metabolism. Flaxseed is full of omega-3 fatty acids, fiber and lignan. Testosterone may be important in the progression of prostate cancer, and lignan in flaxseed binds testosterone cells.[12]

A study at Michigan State University finds that two to four cups of cooked beans a week can lower your risk for heart disease, diabetes and some cancers.[13]

SUGAR FACTS

- Sugar is refined from beets or sugar cane. During the refining process of sugar (made from beets or sugar cane) 100 percent of all nutritional value is removed. You are left with zero nutrients and a lot of calories. Furthermore, when sugar is consumed, it actually robs nutrients from the body, particularly from the teeth and bones. Sugar also is harmful to the stomach lining and can interfere with digestion of nutrients from other food.

- Sugar consumption requires the body to need more nutrients than would otherwise be needed without consuming sugar; therefore, it has been classified by some as an "anti-nutrient."

- Sugar is a drug! It can cause drastic mood swings— from hyperactivity to depression, and has withdrawal symptoms (try to go without it for one day). In addition, the common combination of sugar and starch leads to a fermentation in the digestive process that breaks down to alcohol (a drug) and other toxins.

- When sugar cane is cut it contains about 10-14 percent sucrose. After the refining process, it contains 99.5 percent sucrose! In addition, it is addictive and is used in processed baked goods.

- Americans consume more than 20 teaspoons of sugar a day (320 calories). A can of Pepsi has 10 teaspoons (the USDA recommended daily intake) of sugar and contains 150 calories.

- One teaspoon of sugar (4 grams) has about 16 calories.

- Genuine raw sugar cannot be bought or sold to the general consumer in the United States according to the Food and Drug Administration regulations. All sugar that is bought is in some way refined.

- There is a difference in sugar! In a study conducted in 1937 at the University of Witwatersrand in South Africa, scientists placed thirty-two extracted teeth in water sweetened with refined sugar. After eight weeks fifteen of the teeth had developed cavities. When the same study was done on teeth submerged in unrefined cane juice, only three teeth developed cavities.[14]

- Natural sugars retain vitamins, minerals, and other components essential for their digestion, and are metabolized more slowly than white sugar. White sugar creates a strain on our bodies, depletes stored vitamins and minerals, and suppresses the immune system.

- Chemically, many kinds of sugars exist. Labels could say sucrose, glucose, fructose, maltose, dextrose, lactose, galactose, or levulose. All nutritive sweeteners contain one or more of these sugars.

In view of all its adverse effects on human health, it becomes difficult to defend the common perception of sugar as a food rather than a poison or an addictive drug.

THE WHITE SUGAR MASK

Because of our sweet tooth, and manufacturers' desire to make money, sugar terms have been misleading. "Natural," "whole," and "unrefined" are terms without legal protection. Food companies may use corn sweetener and disguise it, for example, as "raw sugar." In addition, some natural food companies confuse consumers more by implying that these sugars are quality "unrefined" sugar products. These sugars are still separated from the molasses. Some sugar names include:

Brown Sugar
Demerara
Evaporated Cane Juice
Florida Crystals
Muscovado
Naturally Milled Organic Cane Juice
Organic Plantation Milled Sugar
Organic Whole Cane Sugar
Raw Sugar
Sucanat
Turbinado
Unrefined Cane Juice
Whole Cane
Yellow-D

Even if a product is "organic" does not mean it isn't refined.

Some reliable companies use only superior quality sweeteners such as unseparated cane (rapadura), pure maple syrup, malt syrups, fruit juice, or honey (look for raw, organic).

Finally, even if it is a natural sugar—you still need to limit it—or avoid it!

NOTES

THE MORE NUTRIENTS IN YOUR DIET, THE HIGHER YOUR ENERGY LEVEL. THE HIGHER YOUR ENERGY LEVEL, THE MORE EFFICIENT YOUR BODY. THE MORE EFFICIENT YOUR BODY, THE BETTER YOU FEEL AND THE MORE YOU WILL USE YOUR TALENT TO PRODUCE OUTSTANDING RESULTS.

5

WHAT THE BIBLE SAYS ABOUT FOOD

GOD IS THE ultimate Creator. That includes creating food. The nutrients in food are there for a reason. Man has taken something God created to be good and destroyed it. Man has removed vitamins, minerals, and other nutrients. In addition, our foods have been sprayed with pesticides, hormones, drugs, antibiotics—and layered with additives. Due to man's focus on wealth and not health, the soil is not properly fertilized with organic matter and minerals.

The food mentioned in the Bible is unadulterated and natural. Most food consumed today has been altered from God's original design. Our food has been so significantly altered that it is no longer healthy. I urge you to eat the foods in God's natural form. Look for foods that are certified organic, raw, and free of chemicals, preservatives, and additives.

The following foods are hard to find in a raw, natural form so I recommend either eliminating them or eating them in small quantities (special occassions): Dairy products, fish, wild game (meat), and eggs.

Turn from what man has made and get back to what God has made. Here are scriptures that talk about foods. The Bible contains many more scriptures that contain reference to foods. Again, I urge you to read and study for yourself what God says about health.

APPLES

Strengthen me with raisins, refresh me with apples, for I am faint with love. Song of Solomon 2:5, NIV

A word aptly spoken is like apples of gold in settings of silver. Proverbs 25:11, NIV

BARLEY

For the LORD your God is bringing you into a good land—a land with streams and pools of water, with springs flowing in the valleys and hills; a land with wheat and barley, vines and fig trees, pomegranates, olive oil and honey; a land where bread will not be scarce and you will lack nothing; a land where the rocks are iron and you can dig copper out of the hills. Deuteronomy 8:7-9, NIV

So Naomi returned from Moab accompanied by Ruth the Moabitess, her daughter-in-law, arriving in Bethlehem as the barley harvest was beginning. Ruth 1:22, NIV

BEANS

Take wheat and barley, beans and lentils, millet and spelt; put them in a storage jar and use them to make bread for yourself. You are to eat it during the 390 days you lie on your side. Ezekiel 4:9, NIV

Brought bedding and bowls and articles of pottery. They also brought wheat and barley, flour and roasted grain, beans and lentils, honey and curds, sheep, and cheese from cows' milk for David and his people to eat. For they said, "The people have become hungry and tired and thirsty in the desert." 2 Samuel 17:28-29, NIV

BUTTER

So he took butter and milk and the calf which he had prepared, and set it before them; and he stood by them under the tree as they ate. Genesis 18:8, NKJV

BREAD

Take wheat and barley, beans and lentils, millet and spelt; put them in a storage jar and use them to make bread for yourself. You are to eat it during the 390 days you lie on your side. Ezekiel 4:9, NIV

A man came from Baal Shalishah, bringing the man of God twenty loaves of barley bread baked from the first ripe grain, along with some heads of new grain. "Give it to the people to eat," Elisha said. 2 Kings 4:42, NIV

DAIRY

He will eat curds and honey when he knows enough to reject the wrong and choose the right. And because of the abundance of the milk they give, he will have curds to eat. All who remain in the land will eat curds and honey. Isaiah 7:15-22, NIV

EGGS

People complain when there is no salt in their food. And how tasteless is the uncooked white of an egg! Job 6:6, NLT

If a son shall ask bread of any of you that is a father, will he give him a stone? Or if he ask a fish, will he for a fish give him a serpent? Or if he shall ask an egg, will he offer him a scorpion? Luke 11:11-12, KJV

FIGS

They found an Egyptian in a field and brought him to David. They gave him water to drink and food to eat—part of a cake of pressed figs and two cakes of raisins. He ate and was revived, for he had not eaten any food or drunk any water for three days and three nights. 1 Samuel 30:11-12, NIV

FISH

Of all the creatures living in the water of the seas and the streams, you may eat any that have fins and scales. But all creatures in the seas or streams that do not have fins and scales—whether among all the swarming things or among all the other living creatures in the water—you are to detest.

And since you are to detest them, you must not eat their meat and you must detest their carcasses. Anything living in the water that does not have fins and scales is to be detestable to you. Leviticus 11:9-12, NIV

Of all the creatures living in the water, you may eat any that has fins and scales. Deuteronomy 14:9, NIV

They gave him a piece of broiled fish, and he took it and ate it in their presence. Luke 24:42-43, NIV

FRUIT

Fruit trees of all kinds will grow on both banks of the river. Their leaves will not wither, nor will their fruit fail. Every month they will bear, because the water from the sanctuary flows to them. Their fruit will serve for food and their leaves for healing. Ezekiel 47:12, NIV

For the LORD your God is bringing you into a good land—a land with streams and pools of water, with springs flowing in the valleys and hills; a land with wheat and barley, vines and fig trees, pomegranates, olive oil and honey; a land where bread will not be scarce and you will lack nothing; a land where the rocks are iron and you can dig copper out of the hills. Deuteronomy 8:7, NIV

If you enter your neighbor's vineyard, you may eat all the grapes you want, but do not put any in your basket. Deuteronomy 23:24, NIV

Then he gave a loaf of bread, a cake of dates and a cake of raisins to each person in the whole crowd of Israelites, both men and women. And all the people went to their homes. 2 Samuel 6:19, NIV

We remember the fish we ate in Egypt at no cost—also

the cucumbers, melons, leeks, onions and garlic. Numbers 11:5, NIV

Strengthen me with raisins, refresh me with apples, for I am faint with love. Song of Solomon 2:5, NIV

Then he gave a loaf of bread, a cake of dates and a cake of raisins to each person in the whole crowd of Israelites, both men and women. And all the people went to their homes. 2 Samuel 6:19, NIV

We remember the fish we ate in Egypt at no cost—also the cucumbers, melons, leeks, onions and garlic. Numbers 11:5, NIV

GRAPES

When they reached the Valley of Eshcol, they cut off a branch bearing a single cluster of grapes. Two of them carried it on a pole between them, along with some pomegranates and figs. Numbers 13:23, NIV

Noah, a man of the soil, proceeded to plant a vineyard. Genesis 9:20, NIV

Ahab said to Naboth, "Let me have your vineyard to use for a vegetable garden, since it is close to my palace. In exchange I will give you a better vineyard or, if you prefer, I will pay you whatever it is worth." 1 Kings 21:2, NIV

HERBS

The manna was like coriander seed and looked like resin. The people went around gathering it, and then ground it in a handmill or crushed it in a mortar. They cooked it in a pot or made it into cakes. And it tasted like something made with olive oil. When the dew settled on the camp at night, the manna also came down. Numbers 11:7-9, NIV

A jar of wine vinegar was there, so they soaked a sponge in it, put the sponge on a stalk of the hyssop plant, and lifted it to Jesus' lips. When he had received the drink, Jesus said, "It is finished." With that, he bowed his head and gave up his spirit. John 19:29-30, NIV

Cleanse me with hyssop, and I will be clean; wash me, and I will be whiter than snow. Psalm 51:7, NIV

HONEY

But Jonathan had not heard that his father had bound the people with the oath, so he reached out the end of the staff that was in his hand and dipped it into the honeycomb. He raised his hand to his mouth, and his eyes brightened. 1 Samuel 14:27, NIV

Honey and curds, sheep, and cheese from cows' milk for David and his people to eat. For they said, "The people have become hungry and tired and thirsty in the desert." 2 Samuel 17:29, NIV

Then their father Israel said to them, "If it must be, then do this: Put some of the best products of the land in your bags and take them down to the man as a gift—a little balm and a little honey, some spices and myrrh, some pistachio nuts and almonds." Genesis 43:11, NIV

MEAT

Everything that lives and moves will be food for you. Just as I gave you the green plants, I now give you everything. Genesis 9:3, NIV

The LORD said to Moses, "Say to the Israelites: 'Do

not eat any of the fat of cattle, sheep or goats. The fat of an animal found dead or torn by wild animals may be used for any other purpose, but you must not eat it. Anyone who eats the fat of an animal from which an offering by fire may be made to the LORD must be cut off from his people. And wherever you live, you must not eat the blood of any bird or animal. If anyone eats blood, that person must be cut off from his people.'" Leviticus 7:22-27, NIV

"Say to the Israelites: 'Of all the animals that live on land, these are the ones you may eat: You may eat any animal that has a split hoof completely divided and that chews the cud.'" Leviticus 11:2-3, NIV

"This is a lasting ordinance for the generations to come, wherever you live: You must not eat any fat or any blood." Leviticus 3:17, NIV

MELON

We remember the fish we ate in Egypt at no cost—also the cucumbers, melons, leeks, onions and garlic. Numbers 11:5, NIV

The Daughter of Zion is left like a shelter in a vineyard, like a hut in a field of melons, like a city under siege. Isaiah 1:8, NIV

MILK AND CURDS

So I have come down to rescue them from the hand of the Egyptians and to bring them up out of that land into a good and spacious land, a land flowing with milk and honey— the home of the Canaanites, Hittites, Amorites, Perizzites, Hivites and Jebusites. Exodus 3:8, NIV

And because of the abundance of the milk they give, he will have curds to eat. All who remain in the land will eat curds and honey. Isaiah 7:22, NIV

Honey and curds, sheep, and cheese from cows' milk for David and his people to eat. For they said, "The people have become hungry and tired and thirsty in the desert." 2 Samuel 17:29, NIV

You will have plenty of goats' milk to feed you and your family and to nourish your servant girls. Proverbs 27:27, NIV

NUTS

Then their father Israel said to them, "If it must be, then do this: Put some of the best products of the land in your bags and take them down to the man as a gift—a little balm and a little honey, some spices and myrrh, some pistachio nuts and almonds. Genesis 43:11, NIV

OLIVES

Command the Israelites to bring you clear oil of pressed olives for the light so that the lamps may be kept burning. Exodus 27:20, NIV

...until I come and take you to a land like your own, a land of grain and new wine, a land of bread and vineyards, a land of olive trees and honey. Choose life and not death! 2 Kings 18:32a, NIV

ONIONS

We remember the fish we ate in Egypt at no cost—also the cucumbers, melons, leeks, onions and garlic. Numbers 11:5, NIV

POMEGRANATES

A land with wheat and barley, vines and fig trees, pomegranates, olive oil and honey... Deuteronomy 8:8, NIV

SPICES

Woe to you, teachers of the law and Pharisees, you hypocrites! You give a tenth of your spices—mint, dill and cumin. But you have neglected the more important matters of the law—justice, mercy and faithfulness. You should have practiced the latter, without neglecting the former. Matthew 23:23 NIV

Woe to you Pharisees, because you give God a tenth of your mint, rue and all other kinds of garden herbs, but you neglect justice and the love of God. You should have practiced the latter without leaving the former undone. Luke 11:42 NIV

VEGETABLES

"Please test your servants for ten days: Give us nothing but vegetables to eat and water to drink. Then compare our appearance with that of the young men who eat the royal food, and treat your servants in accordance with what you see." So he agreed to this and tested them for ten days. At the end of the ten days they looked healthier and better nourished than any of the young men who ate the royal food. So the guard took away their choice food and the wine they were to drink and gave them vegetables instead. To these four young men God gave knowledge and understanding of all kinds of literature and learning. And Daniel could understand visions and dreams of all kinds. Daniel 1:12-17, NIV

We remember the fish we ate in Egypt at no cost—also the cucumbers, melons, leeks, onions and garlic. Numbers 11:5, NIV

"Take wheat and barley, beans and lentils, millet and spelt; put them in a storage jar and use them to make bread for yourself. You are to eat it during the 390 days you lie on your side. Ezekiel 4:9, NIV

Then God said, "Let the land produce vegetation: seed-bearing plants and trees on the land that bear fruit with seed in it, according to their various kinds." And it was so. Genesis 1:11, NIV

Then God said, "I give you every seed-bearing plant on the face of the whole earth and every tree that has fruit with seed in it. They will be yours for food." Genesis 1:29, NIV

WATER

For the LORD your God is bringing you into a good land of flowing streams and pools of water, with springs that gush forth in the valleys and hills. It is a land of wheat and barley, of grapevines, fig trees, pomegranates, olives, and honey. It is a land where food is plentiful and nothing is lacking. It is a land where iron is as common as stone, and copper is abundant in the hills. Deuteronomy 8:7-9, NIV

WHEAT

But ten of them said to Ishmael, "Don't kill us! We have wheat and barley, oil and honey, hidden in a field." So he let them alone and did not kill them with the others. Jeremiah 41:8, NIV

Take wheat and barley, beans and lentils, millet and spelt; put them in a storage jar and use them to make bread for yourself. You are to eat it during the 390 days you lie on your side. Ezekiel 4:9, NIV

NOTES

Introduction

1. Centers for Disease Control and Prevention web site: <www.cdc.gov/nccdphp/dnpa/obesity/trend/prev_char.htm>. visited on 1/14/05.

2. Centers for Disease Control and Prevention web site: <ww.cdc.gov/nccdphp/sgr/mm.htm.> visited on 1/11/05.

3. Centers for Disease Control and Prevention web site: <www.cdc.gov/nccdphp/overview.htm.> visited on 1/14/05.

PART ONE: Cracking the Code of the Diet Industry

1. Ellen Goodstein, "10 Secrets of the Weight-Loss Industry." Found on web site visited on January 14, 2005: <www.bankrate.com/brm/news/advice/20040113a1.asp>.

Chapter 4

1. Michael F. Jacobson, Ph.D., "Liquid Candy: How Soft Drinks are Harming Americans' Health." Center for Science in the Public Interest web site: <www.cspinet.org/sodapop/liquid_candy.htm.> visited on 1/11/05.

Chapter 5

1. U.S. Food and Drug Administration web site: <www.fda.gov/opacom/backgrounders/foodlabel/newlabel.

html.> visited on 1/11/05.

2. "CSPI'S Guide to Food Additives," Center for Science in the Public Interest web site: <www.cspinet.org/ reports/chemcuisine.htm.> visited on 1/11/05.

Appendix 4

1. Dr. George H. Malkmus and Michael Dye, *God's Way to Ultimate Health: A common sense guide for eliminating sickness through nutrition* (Shelby, N.C.: Hallelujah Acres Publishing 1995), 96.

2. Elizabeth Weise, "Consumers May Have a Beef with Cattle Feed," *USA Today* web site: <www.usatoday.com/ news/health/2003-06-09-beef-cover_x.htm.> visited on 1/14/05.

3. John Fauber, "Is it time to chuck meat? Compelling evidence supports vegetarianism as a hedge against cancer and heart disease," (*Milwaukee Journal Sentinel* staff, March 16, 1997). Found on web site visited on January 14, 2005: <www.geocities.com/RainForest/2062/ chuckmeat.html.>

4. Dr. George H. Malkmus and Michael Dye, *God's Way to Ultimate Health: A common sense guide for eliminating sickness through nutrition* (Shelby, N.C.: Hallelujah Acres Publishing 1995), p. 99.

5. R.B. McLean, "Got Milk and ... Got Osteoporosis? How's that? Doesn't milk protect you from bone loss?" Found on web site visited on January 11, 2005: <www.cyberparent. com/nutrition/osteoporosiscalciumprotein.htm.>

6. Not Milk web site visited on January 11, 2005: <www. notmilk.com/badbones.html.>

7. Not Milk web site visited on January 16, 2005: <www. notmilk.com/deb/092098.html.>

8. Physicians Committee for Responsible Medicine, Milk Does Not Protect Against Bone Breaks Ad, (Spring 1999, Volume VIII, Number 2). Found on web site visited on January 14, 2005: <www.pcrm.org/magazine/ GM99Spring/GM99Spring3.html.>

9. *The Lancet*, (May 8, 1937), 1142. Found on web site visited on January 11, 2005: <www.rawmilk.com.>

10. "Finessing the Flavonoids," published in *Agricultural Research* magazine (February 2001). Found on web site visited on January 15, 2005: <www.ars.usda.gov/is/AR/ archive/feb01/flav0201.htm.>

11. S. Van Duym, Elizabeth Pivonka, *Journal of the American Dietetic Association* (December 2000).

12. Found on web site visited on January 14, 2005: <www. greenleafproduct.com/Prostate_Cancer_Flax_Hull_ Lignan_Benefits.html.>

13. Found on web site visited on January 11, 2005: <www. thebreastsite.com/news/womens-healthy-diet.aspx.>

14. Brigitte Mars, "Like a Kid in A Candy Store". Found on web site visited on January 11, 2005: <www.innerself. com/Health/mars07243.htm.>

"LONG LIFE TO YOU! GOOD HEALTH TO YOU AND YOUR HOUSEHOLD!
AND GOOD HEALTH TO ALL THAT IS YOURS!"
—SAMUEL 25:6 NIV

www.ingramcontent.com/pod-product-compliance
Lightning Source LLC
Chambersburg PA
CBHW020428290526
45785CB00002B/758